Acclaim from health and fitness experts:

"What I like about this book is that it bridges the gap scientifically between the health and fitness researchers, and the lay public. Yet, it effectively manages to satisfy both groups. It's an enjoyable read for anyone looking to take a more active role in improving the many facets of being more active, productive, and feeling better."
  —*Robert H. Gordon, M.S., P.T., M.Ed., Boston, Massachusetts*

"Eat less, sleep more contains time tested science based advice that is hard to argue with; rest the mind and body, exercise moderately and control calorie intake. In our rapid paced and busy environment it is easy to lose sight of these basic guidelines. Dr. Hesslink's book helps us pause and adjust our tempo, just the right prescription for a healthy lifestyle."
  —*Eldon W. Askew, Ph.D., Professor Emeritus, Department of Nutrition and Integrative Physiology, University of Utah*

"This book by Dr. Robert Hesslink provides expert practical advice on important lifestyle choices. Well written and easy to read, the book contains many suggestions that could help you make appropriate choices and enhance your quality of life."
  —*Walter Frontera, M.D., Ph.D., Professor and Chair, Department of Physical Medicine and Rehabilitation, Vanderbilt University Medical Center*

Eat Less, Sleep More, and Slow Down

The science behind healthy living!

Robert Louis Hesslink Jr, ScD

Contents

Introduction

You probably already know that people are living longer. Your Aunt Shirley is closing in on 90 and doesn't appear to be slowing down. But then again, Uncle Harry is in his mid-70's and was just recently admitted to a skilled nursing facility. Some of us may be living longer, but not necessarily living better.

It is important to understand that your health is mostly driven by two factors: genetics and personal choice. Since Frances Crick and James Watson identified the concept of the DNA helix (1), the understanding of genes has increased 1000 fold. The Human Genome Project provided scientists with an understanding of how our lives are controlled by genetic switches (2). At the present time, we may not be able to control or manipulate genes for immortality, but it isn't inconceivable that in the future it may become a reality.

Personal choice is the other factor that drives our health and longevity (3). As I will discuss throughout this book, there are many health problems that are derived from poor choices. It is these that I wish to address in the following pages.

Basically, I believe that there are three health strategies that can help you achieve better health and longevity. These are to *eat less, sleep more and slow down*:

1) *'Eating less' reduces the need for excess energy storage (fat) and increases utilization of circulating and stored stomach and liver fat;*

2) *'Sleeping more' increases day time energy, which reduces the feeling of fatigue, improves memory retention, and helps regulate glucose (sugar) metabolism;*

3) *Aging is a process that is time dependent but influenced by the many facets of your daily life. So, 'slowing down' brings the pace of life more into balance with your daily energy demands and personal responsibilities.*

The concept of eating less and sleeping more sounds nice, but in all reality, it is very difficult to achieve. Try slowing down in this fast-paced, 24/7 world, and you will find yourself without friends and, perhaps, without a job. The global world has brought into play the notion that time is money, why waste it on such simple things as sleep and relaxation? And, with the abundance of food and drink at every corner, why not indulge your sweet tooth along the way?

Sadly, this fast-paced lifestyle along with poor nutrition and low physical activity are the primary factors leading to global obesity and diabetes, whose rates have increased significantly over the past several decades. Obesity and diabetes account for a large share of the world's healthcare expenditures (4). It is estimated that there are 2.1 billion people globally who are overweight and obese with the cost of obesity close to 2.8% of the world's gross domestic product (5).

In the United States, the direct cost associated with diabetes is about $245 billion (6). In addition, it is estimated that the combined costs of being overweight and obese in the United States is close to $1.72 trillion dollars (7).

The point I wish to make is that most of the physiological and bio-chemical changes associated with diabetes and obesity are preventable. Just think about the cost savings to society if we could reduce the incidence of diabetes and obesity on a global scale.

I believe the key for improved global health is for people to engage in a healthier lifestyle with sound decision making in regard to healthy choices pertaining to food, sleep, and relaxation. If people make a concerted effort to improve their health, they can lower their healthcare expenditures, reducing the impact on the healthcare system. But, in order to engage and make an impact, people need to be educated and informed. So, sit back, relax, and enjoy this material. I hope it provides insight and motivation in your quest for better health, better sleep, and a better quality of life.

1

Eat Less

The concept of eating less is not new. In fact, one can imagine the earliest experiences of eating less were common during pre-historic times (8). Whether our ancestors were "hunters or gatherers," their access to daily food sources was probably limited, and it isn't too hard to imagine that they probably trekked around hungry most of the time. While there is no direct record, I suspect that one didn't see many overweight or obese pre-historic residents walking about the landscape in search of food and shelter.

Hunger, in my view, is experienced when the body senses a need for the energy currency, adenosine tri-phosphate (ATP). It is ATP which provides the chemical energy to drive almost every physiological and biochemical process in the body (9). It can be derived from substrates without oxygen for short periods of time, but mostly the production of ATP comes through the use of oxygen on a real time and continuous basis. Needless to say, it is the lack of ATP that generates this hunger signal because, without ATP, death will ensue.

The low energy signal tells the surrounding tissue or organ that something needs to be done. This "something" usually means that more oxygen is needed which results in increased blood flow to the affected tissue—think of a heart attack and the blockage of arteries to the heart tissue. However, the low energy signal can also be a function of reduced substrate delivery. In this case, the substrate(s) in question is glucose, fat and in extreme cases, protein. The cells of our bodies require ATP to function and without energy to replace stored energy, the cell will cease to function adequately and efficiently.

The feeling of hunger is usually driven by changes in energy substrate imbalance due to daily metabolic processes. Energy is derived from primary food sources (protein, fat, and carbohydrates) and is regulated throughout the body by various hormones and metabolic substrates (10). Early research showed that hormones produced by the gut were instrumental in directing the message of satiety or hunger (11). These hormones communicate what is happening inside the stomach and in-testines to the hypothalamus within the brain. It is this feedback system that helps control normal hunger and food intake. It is thought that an imbalance in this feedback system may account for some of the indi-vidual differences in weight control and management.

A state of hunger is usually felt during periods of reduced eating or fast-ing resulting in a low energy state within the cells. We all experience some form of fasting as we sleep at night. After the last meal of the day, our body begins to shift from a fed-state to a fasted-state. Depending upon the circulating level of energy nutrients, it may take hours before the body starts to sense an energy need and express that need as 'hun-ger.' In today's society, except in areas with extreme poverty, most people don't wake up with a ravenous urge to eat. However, if you ex-tend that fasted state into the late morning you just might start to experience symptoms of an energy deficit—growling stomach, light-headedness, and agitation.

Acute hunger is not the same as chronic fasting or starvation. There has been plenty of written evidence outlining the use of fasting or acute star-vation during religious ceremonies (12). Did Moses not fast for forty days and forty nights before he was given the strength to write down the Ten Commandments? And, from Psalms 109:24, it is written, "My knees are weak through fasting; my body has become gaunt, with no fat." There are at least eleven different religions that allow or require some form of fasting. The reasons for such fasting practices run the gamut from "being close to our creator" to "resisting gluttony." In fact, gluttony is considered one of the seven capital sins in the Christian religion. Dante described gluttony as one of the "circles of hell" in his classic poem, "Inferno." Some cultures fast more than others, but fasting has been a common thread across many cultures for thousands of years.

What are the effects of acute fasting and chronic starvation on biological and metabolic parameters?

While there was some research on this topic in the early 1900's, most of the substantive research came from the experiences of World War II prisoners (13). Dr. Ancel Keys, from the University of Minnesota, helped develop the K-ration for American troops during the war. His pioneering research published in his book, *The Biology of Human Starvation,* is still considered to be the best medical textbook on acute and chronic starvation (14). Dr. Keys continued to pursue his interest in diet and health and was instrumental in highlighting the impact of different dietary fats on serum cholesterol and health. In fact, he was on the cover of *Time* magazine in 1961 for his ground-breaking, if not controversial, beliefs. His feeling was that Americans ate too much food, which he discussed at length in his 1963 book, *Eat Well and Stay Well* (15). What he didn't say was that by eating so much as a society, we were taking in excessive calories and, unlike our ancestors, the calories weren't being used by working on the farms and ranches across the country.

The way we eat has been dictated by the circadian nature of our planet for centuries. After a full night's sleep and fasting, our body requires nourishment, both in fluid and energy sources. Before the development of lights, this meal was usually consumed at day break. The men would go off to work the fields, while the women would stay home and care for the children and the house. At midday, the workers needed a chance to rest and re-energize, which meant some kind of meal. As the sun set and daily chores ended, the workers, who were usually family, met for the final meal of the day. While varied in some form or another, this pattern has existed in a wide variety of cultures and communities for centuries.

In looking at your own daily schedule, I am sure you will agree that this historic timetable is a bit outdated for your current lifestyle. Your days are not set by the sun nor the moon. The daily schedule is influenced by many factors that are often out of your control: the kids are late, your boss changed the time of the meeting, or your spouse missed the train. In addition, the role of women in the work force has re-shaped the typical home experience over the past twenty-five years. Now people are asked to fit "three square meals" into that schedule. Good luck with that! It is no wonder that we often fail to achieve sound, nutritional practices consistently.

When we think of dieting or eating less, we have to think about how that can be done most efficiently and effectively. What is the best strategy? Do you stick with three meals a day or should you spread it out? It is no wonder that many times people just give up. It becomes too complex and overwhelming, so the easiest path is to do nothing. But, I am going to show you how to understand the process better, so you can decide what is best for you and your life.

There are many ways to eat less. You can just reduce the calories within each of your meals or you can perhaps eat more meals, but smaller, throughout the day. There is research showing that the use of smaller meals, spread throughout the day, helps reduce late afternoon and evening cravings (16). It really is a matter of choice as to whether you have the standard three square meals or five smaller meals. What matters most is that they are balanced in nutrient content as we will discuss later in the chapter.

Alternate Day Fasting

We talked earlier about the use of fasting as part of a cultural or religious practice. And, there is some new research showing that various strategies of fasting can help reduce body weight and improve health outcomes. One such strategy is the "alternate day of fasting," or ADF approach. In this strategy, an individual is allowed to follow their normal food and beverage schedule but then is required to fast the next day. The severity of fasting can vary depending upon the individual. Research on animals provides a more convincing picture than what has been reported in the limited human clinical trials (17, 18). Varady and Hellerstein (19) reported that the findings in animals suggest that an ADF diet can moderate disease risk factors related to cholesterol and blood pressure, but the story is not so clear in humans.

While the data suggests that an ADF diet might have some benefit, I suspect that, in reality, following such a diet program is difficult. This is true when given the varied schedules at home and work. Just think of having to miss out on the big family birthday gathering or telling your client that you can't eat during your business dinner meeting! It might be a great conversation starter, but perhaps not too conducive for building that business relationship over a shared dining experience.

Intermittent Fasting

Besides fasting on alternate days, there are some newer programs that use intermittent fasting that may be more user friendly. The first, *The 5:2 Diet Book* by Dr. Michael Mosley (20), encourages an individual to eat normally for five days during any given week, and then consume a very low calorie diet for two days (e.g., women—500 calories per day; men—600 calories per day). The essence of this diet program is that it forces you to reduce your caloric intake so that your body will make adjustments in your metabolism and blood sugar regulation. Psychologically, it is believed that by allowing an individual a greater number of normal days, it is much easier to suffer through the fasting days. At the time of this publication, there is only one clinically based study which has documented the physiological and biochemical changes of this type of diet (21). The results showed that after six months, subjects following the 5:2 diet lost appreciable body weight and body fat although the values were not significantly different than a comparative group of women using a normal schedule, low calorie diet.

Another version of the intermittent fasting concept is based on research from the Norris Cancer Center at the University of Southern California. Investigators from USC found that mice undergoing cancer therapy had better clinical outcomes when following an intermittent fasting diet (22). The dietary program (ProLon™) consists of plant-based compounds that are delivered via energy bars, shakes, and soups manufactured by L-Nutra, a company formed by the USC investigators to capitalize on their research (23). Basically, the individuals follow the dietary program for five days and then eat normally for 25 days. As this is an on-going study, it is perhaps too early to say what the success will be. However, without dietary education and exercise, it is hard to imagine that this type of program will induce long lasting benefits.

In addition, it is hard to imagine that an overweight person will respond the same as one who is undergoing very intensive chemotherapy since their metabolic and biochemical profiles are quite different. L-Nutra continues to pursue research into low calorie fasting for weight loss and recently received a grant from the National Institutes of Health to investigate the combination of ingredients in their compound, ChemoLive™, for helping in the fight against obesity. Lee and Longo reviewed the impact of fasting versus dietary restriction on cellular protection and cancer treatment (24). The authors concluded that fasting has the potential to be an effective clinical intervention for patients receiving chemotherapy.

So what really goes on with your body when you eat less?

When we think about weight loss, we usually think about reduced caloric intake both in beverage and food form. Simply said, the three main food forms are fats, proteins, and carbohydrates. These three food components provide the energy that is required to run our physiological and biochemical machinery.

Like gasoline in an automobile, the body needs food, and for the most part, that means carbohydrates which usually take the form of glucose. Glucose is just another term for sugar that we all love and hate. Hopefully, you look at food labels and limit the amount of dietary sugar you consume. But, it is an important energy source that our bodies need in order to function correctly.

Why are carbohydrates so important in the energy process? There are several possible answers, but the one I believe has the strongest science relates to the fact that bacteria developed the system for using carbon-based nutrients for energy during our evolutionary development. As evolutionary processes unfolded, carbon-based resources became abundant, and thus their use became ubiquitous throughout the evolutionary chain. You can see why a daily goal should be the maintenance of a normal blood glucose level. But, remember, unnecessarily high levels of blood glucose cause major health problems, if uncontrolled (25).

Food Intake and Blood Glucose

After a meal, blood glucose rises and the body begins to adjust its level through various mechanisms (26). Foremost is the release of the hormone, insulin, from the pancreas. This hormone is integral for helping glucose enter cells through cell membrane transport. The primary organs for glucose utilization are the liver, brain, and skeletal muscle (27). The liver and skeletal muscle serve as storage deposits for glycogen, the physiologic equivalent of starch. The liver functions at a high energy level because of its function as a metabolic garbage disposal, while skeletal muscle has a constant need due to its structural support and movement functions.

As blood glucose begins to decline, this low energy state causes a great number of enzymatic and biochemical reactions to elevate blood glucose. These include releasing sugar, which is stored as glycogen within the liver and muscle tissues. This cycle of "use-store-use" is what causes many people to fail when it comes to dieting. The term "yo-yo" diet is a common expression and reflects that many people lose weight only to regain it back, and then a little more. Remember, the evolution of the human metabolic regulatory mechanisms came about during periods of very low energy resources, so the tendency to store excess calories is very strong.

Without going into too much detail, chronic starvation is a very unpleasant and unhealthy experience. As the availability of energy from food declines, the body must begin to adapt and adjust in order to maintain adequate blood glucose levels (28). This is done through "gluconeogenesis," which means that fat or protein are converted to sugar at the expense of tremendous amounts of energy consumption (29). In extreme cases, the body starts to scavenge muscle tissue proteins so they can be broken down into amino acids which can then be converted into glucose (14). This is why in chronic starvation you see tremendous muscle wasting.

The point is that one must strive to achieve a balance of low energy intake and high nutrient delivery. Besides the basic fats, proteins, and carbohydrates, the metabolic engine (muscles) needs vitamins, minerals, and various other co-factors in order to function (30).

Caloric restriction is not a new concept, and it has been suggested over the years that pursuing such a lifestyle can extend your life. The majority of the research in this area has been conducted in the research laboratory on mice. In fact, McCay and colleagues (31) first reported on the benefit of caloric restriction on longevity in rats in 1935. There have been numerous studies in mice, flies, fish, and yeast ever since, but there have been very few human clinical trials due to the safety issues related to starvation.

In an attempt to look at large mammalian responses to low caloric intake or starvation, primates have been used in an attempt to replicate the human response to such a challenge. Whether right or wrong, the many studies on primates have provided valuable insights into many of the metabolic diseases and processes that cause a host of problems in humans. The key is to make sure that their sacrifice is humane and beneficial to the understanding of human health (32). There has been some controversy in the field of caloric restriction and longevity. In 2012, the National Institute of Aging reported (33) that there was no benefit of caloric restriction in a controlled primate study, which differed from data reported by the Wisconsin Primate Center (34), which showed significant improvements. While the impact of longevity in primates is still undecided, I believe that the data from each laboratory shows considerable improvement in many cardiovascular and lipid parameters following a calorie restricted diet.

One can imagine that not many individuals would volunteer to be starved, but surprisingly, or perhaps not, there is a dedicated group that follows a very rigid calorie restricted diet. This group, aptly named, the Caloric Restriction Society (CRS), puts into practice what may be considered an extreme version of eating less. The members of this group volunteered for a study conducted by John Holloszy and colleagues (35) out of Washington University in St. Louis, Missouri. This group of men and women were age-matched against a similar group following a standard Western diet and followed for one year. The CRS group exhibited substantial reductions in most parameters associated with morbidity and mortality (e.g., cholesterol, blood pressure, weight).

These findings are consistent with an intervention study conducted by Heilbronn and colleagues (36) at the Pennington Laboratories in Baton Rouge, Louisiana. In this study, non-obese men and women were assigned to either control, caloric restriction (CR), caloric restriction plus exercise or low calorie diet groups. The subjects were to follow this program for six months until they achieved 15% weight reduction and maintenance. Interestingly, the group following the low calorie diet achieved greater weight reduction (13.9%) while the caloric restriction groups lost about 10% each. The control group lost only 1% and neither group was able to achieve the 15% reduction goal over the six months, underscoring the difficulty of weight loss even in the best of environments and situations.

In 2011, Trepanowski and colleagues (18) summarized the available knowledge on caloric restriction diets similar to those found with certain religions. The authors emphasized that no matter how individuals choose to restrict their diet (e.g., daily, alternate day, excluding certain nutrients), there are favorable changes in biomarkers (e.g., cholesterol, lipids, blood pressure) related to cardiovascular and gluco-regulatory function by eating reduced calories.

So what is best for you?

I don't know specifically what "eating less" will mean to you, but it should generally result in a daily lowering of your food intake. A gradual process is more productive than complete starvation due to metabolic regulation and self-preservation processes. Naturally, you should talk with your physician to make sure there are no underlying medical concerns with such a program. However, more than likely they will be happy to hear that you plan on reducing your dietary intake and body weight.

Speaking of body weight, what is the best target or desired body weight? You might want to have this discussion with your health practitioner, or you can get an idea from other sources. First, I believe that most people tend to be at their 'best weight' just out of high school. This usually corresponds with the last growth spurt and before "life" starts to get in the way of daily exercise. Naturally, this might not hold true if you had a weight problem in your younger years, but for most I think it is a good starting point. Next, there are a great number of actuarial tables available on the Internet showing height and weight values for different age brackets. These are used most often in life insurance contracts for determining risk. Be forewarned, the values given are very conservative and in most cases not realistic for most people, nor do they take into account differences related to sports or heavy musculature. However, the standardized tables can give you a good starting point that can be refined later.

Now that you have a good idea of what you think you should weigh or want to weigh, the next part is reducing your dietary intake to help you achieve that goal. There are many dietary formulas, and even smart phone apps, to help determine how many calories to consume on average per day for your age, activity level, and body weight. However, a good estimate is to take your weight and then multiply it by 10. So, if you weigh 110 pounds, your daily energy requirement is approximately 1100 calories. Yes, metabolism is more complex than that, but remember, the more complexity we add to our lives, the less we change.

Once you have established your ideal caloric intake, develop a daily routine to start tracking how many calories you are actually eating. This can be done by pen and paper in a food diary or by an application found on most smart phone platforms. How close are you to this ideal value? If you are above it, then you know what you need to do: eat fewer calories. If you are below it, and yet you still have a hard time losing weight, then it may be time to meet with a health practitioner because there may be hormonal or emotional issues preventing weight loss. But, don't despair—at least now you know you need a little more information and counseling.

Managing your caloric intake doesn't have to be complex. There are a great number of books and blogs that offer advice on various diets and menu planning, so I won't spend time on this topic. In general, one must work towards a balanced diet of fats, proteins, and carbohydrates every day. The fad of high carb or low fat diets has been proven to be less beneficial than just a balanced diet alone (37). Currently, there is great fanfare about the "Paleo" or "caveman" diet. Konoff (38) characterized this diet as containing "wild-animal source and uncultivated-plant source foods, such as lean meat, fish, vegetables, fruits, roots, eggs, and nuts. The diet excludes grains, legumes, dairy products, salt, refined sugar, and processed oils, all of which were unavailable before humans began cultivating plants and domesticating animals." He considered relevant material on the topic in terms of Type II Diabetes prevention and treatment. Dr. Konoff stated that this diet was not necessarily new, but that it had some promise for treating the diabetic patient. Likewise, a study published early this year by Masharani and colleagues out of the University of California, San Francisco reported that in a small sample of patients (n=14), consuming the Paleo diet for 14 days, improved glucose control and lipid profiles when compared to those on a conventional diet (39). The key for the 'eat less' program is to have a balanced diet as outlined by the USDA and other health agencies (40).

Once you decide on a dietary plan, you have to be realistic about what kind of weight loss you can achieve. As shown on "The Biggest Loser" reality show, people can make phenomenal improvements to their health. Granted, these are extreme examples and often are achieved through very special programs, counseling, and include financial incentive. But, the point is that you can achieve significant improvements with discipline and patience. You also have to be realistic about what you can achieve. A large framed person will not become a healthy looking "skinny girl" model but can be a very healthy and fit large person.

The easiest way to record and track your progress is by using a standard bathroom scale. Yes, there are other options, which we will discuss, but for the most part, keeping track of your body weight this way is simple and cost-effective. There are some great new health programs and applications for mobile phones and tablets that can help you track calories, food consumption, food nutrients and body weight.

For a little better measure of body health assessment, it has become standard to use the body mass index (BMI) developed by Adolphe Quetelet in 1832 (41). BMI is the ratio of weight to height and is fairly predictive of health and longevity. The range of BMI's from the Centers for Disease Control can be used as guidelines—Normal is 18.5 to 24.9;

Overweight is 25 to 29.9; and Obese is 30 and above (42). See the link in Chapter 4.

Body composition is different than BMI in that it is a reflection of how much fat mass you carry as a percentage of your overall body mass. The gold standard for determining body composition is based on the work of Archimedes and his displacement theory for objects submersed in water (43). Basically, fat is more buoyant than muscle, which leads to a lower body density when calculated by standard formulas. Generally, women tend to have a higher percentage of body fat due to maternal requirements. Gallagher and colleagues (44) provided predictive guidelines for body fat composition in a study using dual energy x-ray absorption (DEXA) methodology. The range of average body fat percentage in women was 21% to 43% and in men between 8% and 30%. While everyone can easily calculate BMI, it is not so easy to get body composition through underwater weighing. However, body fat can be determined through a variety of other methods as reviewed by Wells and Fewtrell (45). These authors discuss the merits of skinfold calipers and body impedance assessment which are commonly available at sports clubs and health clinics. The key is to use a methodology that is convenient and affordable for you.

You Got to "Move It, Move It"

It is important that you perform some daily physical activity. The ability to experience life changing weight loss and maintenance through diet alone is virtually impossible. If skeletal muscle is the main structure of our metabolic engine, then we need to use it regularly. Plain and simple—muscle helps burn circulating energy (e.g., sugar and fat), releases stored energy and I believe keeps everything in tip-top shape. How you move is up to you, but there are guidelines that should be implemented into your daily schedule. The American College of Sports Medicine (ACSM) recommends the following guideline in order to achieve physical activity and weight loss success (46):

Adults should participate in at least 150 minutes/week of moderate-intensity physical activity to prevent significant weight gain and reduce associated chronic disease risk factors. For most adults, this amount of physical activity can be easily achieved in 30 minutes/day, five days a week. Overweight and obese individuals will most likely experience greater weight reduction and prevent weight regain with 250+ minutes/week of moderate-intensity physical activity. ACSM also recommends strength training as part of this health and fitness regimen, in order to increase fat-free mass and further reduce health risks.

Once you have determined your body weight goal, it is time to start lowering your caloric intake to meet that daily caloric requirement needed for your body weight. Remember, as outlined above, your body has a built-in system to conserve energy, when it senses that the energy balance is out of range. So you must be careful not to shut down the metabolic machine when embarking on your weight loss plan. The American College of Sports Medicine (ACSM) recommends that overweight and obese individuals reduce their current energy (calorie) intake by 500 to 1,000 kcals per day to achieve weight loss (47). Basically, to meet this goal, all you need to do is cut out one fruit smoothie, iced coffee drink or hamburger from your diet, which doesn't seem all that difficult once you think about it—right?

If you find the ACSM recommendation difficult to achieve, I suggest reducing your daily caloric intake by 15% increments for women and 25% for men. For example, if a woman weighs 150 pounds, her maintenance daily intake should be around 1500 calories. To determine the daily calories required to help lose weight, take her maintenance intake of 1500 times 0.85 to get 1275 calories. The goal is to be able to consume this amount of calories (e.g., 1275) without feeling hungry or having the urge to snack. This is where mental discipline, small snacks throughout the day, and the use of high density, low calorie foods come into play.

In full disclosure, there is no published data on this reduction level, but I believe it is something that most people can achieve consistently and with good results. Naturally, your results may vary and, as always, check with your health practitioner before attempting any fitness or weight loss program.

How Long Before You See Results

Do you have a cousin that can eat anything and stay slim? Or, perhaps a friend who joined a gym with you, but now looks incredible after just two weeks, and you look, well, the same? Annoying, I know, but these examples just highlight that we are all individuals with different levels of metabolism, discipline, and underlying hormonal differences. The best advice is to be happy for them, but don't let their progress get in the way of your progress. What matters is how you look when you hit your number!

Being active by following the ACSM guidelines will help you get to your goal. But, I suggest staying on your new low-caloric schedule for at least 21 days depending upon how your body responds. This is where the weekly tracking of body weight comes in handy because healthy weight loss is excruciatingly slow. When you have achieved your initial body weight goal, then take your new body weight and reduce it again using the appropriate reduction rate (15% or 25%) until you have reached your 'desired' final target body weight. The result of this slow, stepped process is to let your body adjust naturally to fewer calories.

In a recent study published in the *Journal of the American Medical Association (JAMA)*, Johnston and colleagues (48) looked at over 59 research articles related to some kind of diet program. What they found was that most diet programs achieve the same level of body weight loss and general health benefit. However, they all experienced problems preventing the participants from regaining their weight back upon cessation of the given diet. The authors concluded that while diet programs help people lose weight, pharmacological intervention might be useful for helping

19

patients maintain the weight loss. While this may have some merit, I believe that there are better alternatives for helping patients feel satiated than altering their brain chemistry. Fragala and colleagues (49) showed that the use of dietary fiber helped college age women lose body fat and body weight when compared to those consuming placebo. Study participants were not followed after the program, so it is unclear whether the use of dietary fiber provided continued weight loss or maintenance. However, further research by Islam and colleagues (50) suggested that the changes in body weight and circulating hormones induced by similar dietary fibers was directly related to a change in muscle and liver fat oxidation, resulting in an increase in basal metabolism. If energy intake is maintained or even reduced, then these small increases in energy utilization will reduce body fat storage and body weight over time.

The simplicity of dietary fiber for weight loss was examined by Ma and colleagues at the University of Massachusetts Medical School (51). In a published study, participants using a simple diet directing them to eat more fiber from a variety of food sources experienced almost as much weight loss (4.6 vs 6.0 pounds over 12 months) as those following the more rigid guideline from the American Heart Association (52). Ma and colleagues indicated that for some individuals, a more simplified program would be a better alternative, but that it was quite evident that increasing dietary fiber as prescribed by the AHA guidelines provided benefits to not only body weight but lowered blood pressure, and most indices related to diabetes.

Peer to Peer Motivation

The one salient feature that I find of most benefit for any strategy is the use of peer-to-peer interaction and group education (53). This is the basis for programs like Weight Watchers®, Jenny Craig®, and Nutrisystem®, separate from their pre-packaged meals. I don't think the use of support individuals or groups can be emphasized enough when trying to achieve weight management success. Whether through traditional health coaching or mentoring, the use of an outside force to help one achieve success and push beyond personal limits can mean the difference between success and failure. So don't be afraid, ask a friend to go for a walk, or ask that gym rat (male or female) for a few pointers. One thing I know about healthy people is that they love to talk and love to help others.

It is important during this process to start changing your views regarding good healthy, nutritional practices. Given the advent of healthy menus, juice bars, juicing machines, and nutritious foods, it is so much easier than in days past. Once you buy into the notion of healthy eating and living, maintaining a healthy weight will come naturally. Remember, the goal of *Eating Less* is about obtaining and maintaining a desirable body weight for a healthier lifestyle and better long-term survival.

In conclusion, the concept of eating less relates to understanding what good eating and good nutrition means, as well as, the importance of reducing your daily caloric intake. How you achieve this goal is really dependent upon you! There are plenty of examples on TV, in magazines, and in scientific papers that show when an individual decides to become healthy, anything is possible. Why not become one of those examples—for you, your family and your friends?

Simple things you can do:

- Take your time eating, don't rush a meal.
- Share a meal with a friend or significant other.
- Eat half a meal and take the rest home when eating out.
- Wear smaller pants or a tighter belt to make you feel uncomfortable while eating.
- Have a friend help you stay on task and target in meeting your goals.
- Eat smaller meals throughout the day.
- Walk just a little extra each day, then include some weight resistance exercises to help build muscle mass and maintain strength with aging.

Cited References

1. Watson, J. D., & Crick, F. H. C. (1953). A structure for deoxyribose nucleic acid. *Nature, 171*, 737-738.

2. Lander, E. S., Linton, L. M., Birren, B., Nusbaum, C., Zody, M. C., et al. (2001). Initial sequencing and analysis of the human genome. *Nature, 409*(6822), 860-921.

3. Carey, J. R. (2003). *Longevity: The biology and demography of life span.* Princeton, NJ: Princeton University Press.

4. Withrow, D., & Alter, D. A. (2011). The economic burden of obesity worldwide: a systematic review of the direct costs of obesity. *Obesity Reviews, 12*(2), 131–141.

5. Dobbs, R., Sawers, C., Thomson, F., Manyika, J., Woetzel, J., Child, P., Mckenna, S., & Spatharou, A. (2014). *Overcoming obesity: an initial economic analysis.* Retrieved from McKinsey Global Institute website: http://www.mckinsey.com/insights/economic_studies/how_the_world _could_better_fight_obesity

6. American Diabetes Association (2013). Economic costs of diabetes in the U.S. in 2012. *Diabetes Care.* doi: 10.2337/dc12-2625

7. Tsai, A. G., Williamson, D. F., & Glick, H. A. (2011). Direct medical cost of overweight and obesity in the United States: A quantitative systematic review. *Obesity Reviews: An Official Journal of the International Association for the Study of Obesity, 12*(1), 50–61.

8. Mannino, M. A. et al. (2012). Origin and diet of the prehistoric hunter-gatherers on the mediterranean island of favignana (Ègadi Islands, Sicily). Ed. Luca Bondioli. *PLoS ONE, 7*(11): e49802. doi: 10.1371/journal.pone.0049802

9. Parpura, V., Schousboe, A., & Verkhratsky, A. (2014). *Glutamate and ATP at the interface of metabolism and signaling in the brain.* Switzerland: Springer International.

10. Hargreaves, M., & Richter, E. A. (1988). Regulation of skeletal muscle glycogenolysis during exercise. *Canadian Journal of Applied Sport Sciences, 13*(4), 197-203.

11. Parker, H. E., Gribble, F. M., & Reimann, F. (2014). The role of gut endocrine cells in control of metabolism and appetite. *Experimental Physiology, 99*(9), 1116-1120.

12. Beliefnet.com, accessed at http://www.beliefnet.com/Faiths/2001/02/Fasting-Chart.aspx

13. Consolazio, C., Frank, M., Leroy O., Johnson, H. L., Nelson, R. A., & Krzywicki, H. J. (1967). Metabolic aspects of acute starvation in normal humans (10 Days). *The American Journal of Clinical Nutrition, 20,* 672-683.

14. Keys, A., Brozek, J., Henschel, A., Mickelsen, O., & Taylor, H. L. (1950). *The biology of human starvation.* Minneapolis, MN: The University of Minnesota Press.

15. Keys, A., & Keys, M. (1959). *Eat well and stay well.* New York, NY: Doubleday.

16. Mattson, M. P., Allison, D. B., Fontana, L., Harvie, M., Longo, V. D. et al. (2014). Meal frequency and timing in health and disease. *Proceedings of the National Academy of Sciences, 111,* 16647-16653.

17. Hempenstall, S., Picchio, L., Mitchell, S. E., Speakman, J. R., & Selman, C. (2010). The impact of acute calorie restriction on the metabolic phenotype in male C57BL/6 and DBA/2 mice. *Mechanisms of Ageing and Development, 131,* 111-118.

18. Trepanowski, J. F., Canale, R. E., Marshall, K. E., Kabir, M. M. & Bloomer, R. J. (2011). Impact of caloric and dietary restriction regimens on markers of health and longevity in humans and animals: a summary of available findings. *Nutrition Journal, 10,* 107.

19. Varady, K. A. & Hellerstein, M. K. (2007). Alternate-day fasting and chronic disease prevention: a review of human and animal trials. *The American Journal of Clinical Nutrition, 86,* 7-13.

20. Mosley, M., & Spencer, M. (2013). *The fast diet.* New York, NY: Atria Paperback/Simon and Schuster.

21. Harvie, M. N., Pegington, M., Mattson, M. P., Frystyk, J., Dillon, B., et al. (2011). The effects of intermittent or continuous energy restriction on weight loss and metabolic disease risk markers: a randomized trial in young overweight women. *International Journal of Obesity. 35,* 714-717.

22. Fontana, L., Partridge, L., & Longo, V. D. (2010). Extending healthy life space—from yeast to humans. *Science, 328,* 321-326.

23. Prolon, L-Nutra, Inc. Retrieved from http://www.l-nutra.com/index.php/products

24. Lee, C., & Longo, V. D. (2011). Fasting vs dietary restriction in cellular protection and cancer treatment: from model organisms to patients. *Oncogene, 30,* 3305–3316.

25. Kawahito, S., Kitahata, H., & Oshita, S. (2009). Problems associated with glucose toxicity: role of hyperglycemia-induced oxidative stress. *World Journal of Gastroenterology, 15*(33), 4137–4142.

26. Blaak, E. E. et al. (2015). Impact of postprandial glycaemia on health and prevention of disease. *Obesity Reviews, 13*(10), 923–984.

27. O'Neill, H. M. (2013). AMPK and exercise: glucose uptake and insulin sensitivity. *Diabetes & Metabolism Journal, 37*(1), 1–21.

28. Tesfaye, N., & Seaquist, E. R. (2010). Neuroendocrine responses to hypoglycemia. *Annals of the New York Academy of Sciences, 1212,* 12–28.

29. Rui, L. (2014). Energy metabolism in the liver. *Comprehensive Physiology, 4*(1), 177–197.

30. U.S. Department of Agriculture. (2015). *Dietary guidelines for Americans 2015.* Retrieved from http://www.health.gov/dietaryguidelines/2015.asp

31. McCay, C. M., Crowell, M. F., & Maynard, L. A. (1935). The effect of retarded growth upon length of lifespan and upon ultimate body size. *Journal of Nutrition, 10,* 63–79.

32. Tardif, S. D., Coleman, K., Hobbs, T. R., & Lutz, C. (2013). IACUC review of nonhuman primate research. *ILAR Journal, 54*(2). doi:10.1093/ilar/ilt040

33. Mattison, J. A., Roth, G. S., Beasley, T. M., Tilmont, E. M., Handy, A. M., et al. (2012). Impact of caloric restriction on health and survival in rhesus monkeys from the NIA study. *Nature, 489,* 318-321.

34. Colman, R. J., Beasley, T. M., Kemnitz, J. W., Johnson, S. C., Weindruch, R. & Anderson, R. M. (2014). Calorie restriction reduces age-related and all-cause mortality in rhesus monkeys. *Nature Communications, 5*(3557), 1-5.

35. Holloszy, J. O. & Fontana, L. (2007). Caloric restriction in humans. *Experimental Gerontology, 42*, 709-712.

36. Heilbronn, L. K., de Jonge, L., Frisard, M. I., DeLany, J. P., Larson Meyer, D. E., Rood, J. et al. (2006). Effect of 6-mo. calorie restriction on biomarkers of longevity, metabolic adaptation and oxidative stress in overweight subjects. *The Journal of the American Medical Association, 295*, 1539-1548.

37. Balart, L. A. (2005). Diet options of obesity: fad or famous? *Gastroenterology Clinics of North America, 34*(1), 83-90.

38. Klonoff, D. C. (2009). The beneficial effects of a Paleolithic diet on type 2 diabetes and other risk. *Journal of Diabetes Science and Technology, 3*(6), 1229-1232.

39. Masharani, U., Sherchan, P., Schloetter, M., Stratford, S., Xiao, A., Sebastian, A., Nolte, K.M., & Frassetto, L. (2015). Metabolic and physiologic effects from consuming a hunter-gatherer (Paleolithic)-type diet in type 2 diabetes. *European Journal of Clinical Nutrition, 69*(8), 944-948.

40. Haddad, L., Achadi, E., Bend,ch, M. A., Ahuja, A. et al. (2015). The global nutrition report 2014: actions and accountability to accelerate the world's progress on nutrition. *Journal of Nutrition, 145*(4), 663-671.

41. Eknoyan, G. (2008). Adolphe Quetelet (1796-1874)—the average man and indices of obesity. *Nephrology Dialysis Transplantation, 23*(1), 47-51.

42. Centers for Disease Control and Prevention. *Healthy weight – it's not a diet, it's a lifestyle!* Retrieved from http://www.cdc.gov/healthyweight/assessing/bmi/

43. Francis, K. T. (1990). Body-composition assessment using underwater weighing techniques. *Physical Therapy, 70*(10), 657-62.

44. Gallagher, D., Heymsfield, S. B., Heo, M., Jebb, S. A., Murgatroyd, P. R., & Sakamoto,Y. (2000). Healthy percentage body fat ranges: an approach for developing guidelines based on body mass index. *American Journal of Clinical Nutrition, 72*(3), 694-701.

45. Wells, J. C., & Fewtrell, M. S. (2006). Measuring body composition. *Archives of Disease in Childhood, 91*(7), 612-617.

46. Garber, C. E., Blissmer, B., Deschenesm M., Franklin, B. et al. (2011). Quantity and quality of exercise for developing and maintaining cardiorespiratory, musculoskeletal, and neuromotor fitness in apparently healthy adults: guidance for prescribing exercise. *Medicine & Science in Sports & Exercise, 43*(7), 1334-1359.

47. Jakicic, J. M., Clark, K., Coleman, E., Donnelly, J. E., Foreyt, J., Melanson, E., Volek, J., & Volpe, S. L. (2001). American College of Sports Medicine position stand. Appropriate intervention strategies for weight loss and prevention of weight regain for adults. *Medicine & Science in Sports & Exercise, 33*(12), 2145-2156.

48. Johnston, B. C., Kanters, S., Bandayrel, K., Wu, P., Naji, F., Siemieniuk, R. A. et al. (2014). Comparison of weight loss among named diet programs in overweight and obese adults: a meta-analysis. *The Journal of the American Medical Association, 312,* 923-933.

49. Fragala, M. S., Kraemer, W. J., Volek, J. S., Maresh, C. M., Puglisi, M. J., Vingren, J. L., Ho, J. Y., Hatfield, D. L., Spiering, B. A., Forsythe, C. E., Thomas, G. A., Quann, E. E., Anderson, J. M., & Hesslink, R. L. Jr. (2009). Influences of a dietary supplement in combination with an exercise and diet regimen on adipocytokines and adiposity in women who are overweight. *European Journal of Applied Physiology, 105*(5), 665-672.

50. Islam, A., Civitarese, A. E., Hesslink, R. L., & Gallaher, D. D. (2012). Viscous dietary fiber reduces adiposity and plasma leptin and increases muscle expression of fat oxidation genes in rats. *Obesity (Silver Spring), 20,* 349-355.

51. Ma, Y., Olendzki, B. C., Wang, J., Persuitte, G. M, et al. (2015). Single-component versus multi-component dietary goals for the metabolic syndrome: A randomized trial. *Annals of Internal Medicine, 162,* 248-257.

52. Krauss RM, Eckel RM (Eds). (2000). Revision 2000: A statement for healthcare professionals from the nutrition committee of the American Heart Association. *Circulation, 102,* 2284-2299.

53. Dutton, G. R., Phillips, J. M., Kukkamalla, M., Cherrington, A. L., & Safford, M. M. (2015). Pilot study evaluating the feasibility and initial outcomes of a primary care weight loss intervention with peer coaches. *Diabetes Education.* Advance online publication. pii: 0145721715575356

Additional Sources

Barrows, K., & Snook, J. T. (1987). Effect of a high-protein, very-low-calorie diet on resting metabolism, thyroid hormones, and energy expenditure of obese middle-aged women. *The American Journal of Clinical Nutrition, 45,* 391-398.

Brockman, D. A., Chen, X., & Gallaher, D. D. (2012). Hydroxypropyl methylcellulose, a viscous soluble fiber, reduces insulin resistance and decreases fatty liver in Zucker diabetic fatty rats. *Nutrition & Metabolism.* Retrieved from http://www.nutritionandmetabolism.com

Burcelin, R. (2012). Regulation of metabolism: A cross talk between gut microbiota and its human host. *Physiology, 27,* 300.

Cantó, C., & Auwerx, J. (2011). Calorie restriction: Is AMPK a key sensor and effector? *Physiology, 26,* 214.

Davies, H. J., Baird, I.M., Fowler, J., Mills, I. H., Baillie, J. E., Rattan, S., & Howard, A. N. (1989). Metabolic response to low- and very-low-diets. *The American Journal of Clinical Nutrition, 49*(5), 745-751.

Gallaher, C. M., Munion, J., Hesslink, R., Wise, J., Gallaher, D. D. (2000). Cholesterol reduction by glucomannan and chitosan is mediated by changes in cholesterol absorption and bile acid and fat excretion in rats. *The Journal of Nutrition, 130,* 2753-2759.

Haufe, S., Haas, V., Wolfgang, U., Birkenfeld, A. L., Jeran, S., et al. (2013). Long-lasting improvements in liver fat and metabolism despite body weight regain after dietary weight loss. *Diabetes Care, 36,* 3786-3792.

Heilbronn, L. K., & Ravussin, E. (2003). Calorie restriction and aging: review of the literature and implications for studies in humans. *The American Journal of Clinical Nutrition, 78,* 361-369.

Kalsbeek, A., La Fleur, S., Fliers, E. (2014). Circadian control of glucose metabolism. *Molecular Metabolism, 3,* 372-383.

Kluger, J. (2007, May). The science of appetite. *TIME.* Retrieved from http://www.time.com

Larson, D. E., Hesslink, R. L., Hrovat, M. I., Fishman, R. S., Systrom, D. M. (1994). Dietary effects on exercising muscle metabolism and performance by 31P-MRS. *Journal of Applied Physiology, 77,* 1108-1115.

Levitsky, D. A., & Pacanowski, C. R. (2011). Free will and the obesity epidemic. *Public Health Nutrition, 15,* 126-141.

Mănălăchioae, R., Sarpataki, O., Prodan, I., Sevastre, B., & Marcus, I. (2011). The influence of different levels of acute calorie restriction on several hematological and biochemical parameters in Wistar rats. *Veterinary Medicine, 1,* 207-212.

Poole, D. C. & Henson, L. C. (1988). Effect of acute caloric restriction on work efficiency. *The American Journal of Clinical Nutrition, 4,* 15-18.

Purcell, K., Sumithran, P., Prendergast, L. A., Bouniu, C. J., Delbridge, E., & Proietto, J. (2014). The effect of rate of weight loss on long-term weight management: a randomized controlled trial. *The Lancet: Diabetes & Endocrinology, 2,* 954-962.

Speakman, J. R., Levitsky, D. A., Allison, D. B., Bray, M. S, de Castro, J. M., et al. (2011). Set points, settling points and some alternative models: theoretical options to understand how genes and environments combine to regulate body adiposity. *Disease Models and Mechanisms, 4,* 733-745.

Speakman, J. R. (2014). If body fatness is under physiological regulation, then how come we have an obesity epidemic? *Physiology, 29,* 88-98.

Van Horn, L. (2014). A diet by any other name is still about energy. *The Journal of the American Medical Association, 319,* 900-901.

2
Sleep More

Who doesn't want to sleep more, right?

I mean, who hasn't woken up wishing they could just turn off that alarm and go back to sleep? How about during the weekend? You know—a day with no soccer or baseball game, no ballet or karate, no weekend work projects—a real morning to just sleep in.

What is that like? Do you remember…just laying there and slowly becoming conscious of your surroundings…hearing the clock ticking, the kids giggling, or the birds chirping> How did that feel? Great! Didn't it?

When one wakes in this manner, the various systems of the body just start turning on, like your computer booting up—the eyes open, the ears tune in, and the nose might smell freshly brewed coffee or breakfast. You might lay there for a short period, but eventually you rise, and you are ready to start the day. Not rushed, not tired, ready to go— refreshed.

Why can't we experience that every day? Well, you can! No one is stopping you, except society, and perhaps, your family. In order to achieve such an experience requires a serious change in your family and work lifestyle. Our society is not built on this slow morning framework, but instead it is a 24/7, 100-mile-an-hour society. The information we consume every day is overwhelming. And, I do mean consume voraciously. The old saying, "food for thought," has really become a bountiful harvest and takes a toll on our capacity to slow down and enjoy life. Think about it—how many times have you looked at your mobile phone since reading this section? One time? Ten times? What is it that you are looking for—a text from your boss, from your girlfriend or, perhaps, that breaking news story or stock quote?

The term "popcorn brain" was coined by Dr. David Levy from the University of Washington Information School during an interview on CNN with Elizabeth Cohen (1). Basically, popcorn brain defines people whose brain "has become so accustomed to the constant stimulation of electronic multitasking that we're unfit for life offline, where things pop at a much slower pace." You know what I'm talking about—it used to be checking your email, and then text messages and now every notification that is pushed to your smart phone. In reality, the short-burst pattern of notifications and text messages retards the ability for people to maintain focus for long periods.

I opened this section with the notion of you slowly waking up to your own rhythm or cycle. It has been known for quite some time that we all have different cycles relating to sleep, metabolism, hormones, and energy. The circadian clock that regulates the sleep-wake cycle is located in nerve cells within the center of the brain (2). These cells secrete proteins which have a 24-hour biochemical lifespan. These proteins activate receptors within the center of the brain, called the hypothalamus, which controls a large number of standard processes in all mammalians, to sleep and achieve wakefulness (3).

There is a second process within the brain that serves as a feedback mechanism to increase the drive for sleep. It is thought that one of the chemical components of this system is adenosine (4). Adenosine is a secondary by-product of the metabolic breakdown of ATP, the energy currency mentioned in Chapter 1. Adenosine increases due to the metabolic activity during wakefulness, which then serves as negative feedback, resulting in the drive to sleep.

It is widely known that a number of factors inhibit sleep. Of these, caffeine (5) is a very strong inhibitor as well as certain medications (6). These compounds are known to impact adenosine through inhibitory pathways. In order to sleep more and sleep better, one must get a better handle on the timing and consumption of these "sleep inhibitors."

Remember my earlier passage about waking to your own rhythm or circadian clock? Well, a group of students at Brown University took it upon themselves to document the impact of an individual waking naturally. In other words, they wanted to understand what would happen if a person just woke up when their body said it was time to get up, not when the alarm clock told them to get up. They exploited new microtechnology for measuring brain waves and developed a data collection algorithm for analyzing sleep wave patterns. They eventually shifted away from the "wake on your own schedule" idea and concentrated on helping individuals understand their sleep. Their system measured how long it took for a person to fall asleep, how many times they woke up at night, and how many phases of sleep they experienced during the night.

They formed a company, Zeo™, and took advantage of the direct-to-consumer trend. This provided individuals the opportunity to determine the quality of their sleep at home, and it provided the company access to thousands of data points from individuals who uploaded their data every day to Zeo's servers. Shambroom and colleagues (7) from Zeo conducted a study comparing the wireless system (WS) with a traditional polysonograph (PSG) and an actigraph (ACT) in a sleep laboratory. Twenty-nine healthy subjects (a mix of males and females) underwent concurrent assessment on two separate nights. They found that the WS had good agreement with PSG data collected that same night. These findings were corroborated in a later study conducted by

31

Tonetti and colleagues (8) in eleven female volunteers comparing WS and PSG. Basically, what they found was that the Zeo home device could provide sleep data, just as good as those expensive sleep centers.

How much value and benefit the consumers received from this information is unknown. From the testimonials and the published research, it does suggest that having information about sleep can be beneficial to some. I tried Zeo myself and found that the headband containing the electronics was a bit cumbersome and awkward at night. The information about my sleep was interesting, but I really couldn't see a way to incorporate it into a sleep strategy, which may explain why their business model eventually failed.

Whether the do-it-yourself sleep management concept was ill-conceived or ill-timed, the effort by those involved with Zeo should be applauded for being early innovators in the "quantified self" culture.

Sleep and the Quantified Self

The "Quantified Self" is a term for individuals that have embraced the use of new technology for tracking their daily, if not hourly, physiological and biomechanical parameters (9). The ability to manufacture devices with improved electronic fidelity and power usage in wearable form has fueled this movement. While previously the domain of Olympic caliber athletes or military personnel, these newer devices have allowed the weekend athlete to track and achieve performance improvement at a fraction of the cost. Think about pedometers or those expensive Polar heart rate monitors of the past. Pedometers are just simple mechanical devices that measure changes in your hip movement while walking. Polar heart rate monitors were one of the first attempts to use micro-electronics for picking up the electrical signal generated with each heartbeat. Nowadays, products from FitBit®, Jawbone® and Garmin®, serve to function in a similar manner. These devices count changes in motion through electrical pulses embedded inside a small accelerometer. The data can be uploaded to software that helps one analyze and track physical activity.

I believe there is great value in knowing the biometrics of one's health, but I am not certain that the "quantified self" is for everyone. There is a fine line between using information to help guide behavior versus becoming consumed by the information. Information regarding your body weight, sleep, blood cholesterol patterns, and such are vitally important. However, to dwell on such matters minute-by-minute is perhaps over-kill in my opinion.

So what are the stages of sleep?

The standard sleep laboratory device is a 12-lead electroencephalograph (EEG) which measures brain waves during sleep (10). The brain goes through a series of stages that vary in cycle and length. One of the early hallmarks of sleep research was the linkage between brain wave forms and rapid eye movement (11). The two stages of most importance are rapid eye movement (REM) and non-REM sleep.

Non-REM sleep is more of a transitional period that sets the brain and body up for the coming REM sleep (12). For the most part non-REM is not much different from wakefulness. The brain goes through a series of deeper and deeper phases (four to be exact) during non-REM, although the exact reason is unknown.

REM sleep is evidenced by intense rapid eye movement, which some liken to a video playback of the day's events or dreams. However, one big difference is that during REM sleep the brain sends inhibitory signals to the muscles, virtually making the individual paralyzed. This may be a protective process as we know the muscle groups for the heart, lungs, smooth muscles, and diaphragm remain active. Have you ever been jolted out of bed dreaming about kicking a ball, falling down, or trying to protect yourself? You can be assured that was non-REM sleep.

Sleep is very cyclic in nature as the brain goes through non-REM and REM patterns. The amount of time spent in each stage varies per individual but plays an integral role in the sleep quality of that individual (13).

Non-REM is associated with early portions of the sleep cycle, while REM is most often experienced towards the mid and ending phases.

Early researchers considered sleep to be passive and without any major influence on the general physiology or brain function, but sleep is a very active and dynamic process (14). However, it is now known that a great number of important physiological events occur during this period. While sleep has always been viewed as being restorative, current research suggests there is a great deal more to sleep than ever imagined. Major changes in circulating hormones, kidney function, digestion, thermal regulation, and protein synthesis happen while one is sleeping.

Several reports have shown that short duration sleep (< 7 hours per night) leads to dysregulation of appetite (15). Moreover, there is some suggestion in animals that changes in hormones due to sleep disturbance cause a reduction in total energy expenditure. Body energy storage fits a simple equation through the law of thermodynamics—energy in equals energy out. "Energy in" refers to calories consumed, while "energy out" means how much energy is used to support physiological function (e.g., heart, nerves, brain), daily movement, and physical activity. Naturally, a balanced equation means these two components are equal. If we see a shift toward lower energy expenditure as a function of inadequate sleep, then without controlling for energy in, there will be more energy for storage and this storage takes the form of fat. This starts that slow cycle of weight gain because without some intervention, this unhealthy cycle will ultimately take a toll on health and longevity.

Sleep and Glucose Regulation

There is also accumulating evidence that changes in sleep alter blood glucose regulation (16). Remember, glucose is maintained within a narrow range through the effect of insulin and glucagon. It is the major driver of energy for the brain and muscles. It is the interaction between insulin and muscle receptors that encourages the entry of glucose into the muscle for use within the energy pathway to produce ATP (17).

It is well known that diabetics suffer from dysregulation of glucose (18). Type II Diabetes usually occurs in older individuals, who, due to unhealthy lifestyle or perhaps poor genetics, lose the sensitivity for insulin to activate the skeletal transport of glucose. Thus, due to this insensitivity to insulin, the circulating glucose does not enter the muscle and rises in concentration. As we discussed before, high levels of glucose cause toxicity in a number of organs. Thankfully, these alterations in insulin sensitivity can be reversed through the use of exercise and diet (19), often with little or no pharmacological intervention.

It has been reported that reductions in insulin sensitivity can occur in patients after just two weeks of getting only 5.5 hours of sleep per night (20). This has been reported for a variety of short duration sleep suggesting that sleep has an important role in glucose regulation, along with diet and exercise. It is no wonder that sleep disruption has been linked with incidence of diabetes and obesity. Furthermore, the inability to fall asleep or maintain sleep has been associated with a high probability of developing diabetes (21).

The mechanism(s) of how sleep disturbance alters glucose regulation and metabolic function are complex (22). However, there are several possible pathways that have been proposed. It is known that hormones have circadian patterns, oftentimes reaching their low point during sleep. New information suggests that hormonal release and glucose control is dependent upon specific sleep stages. Short sleep duration means the dysregulation of non-REM and REM cycling such that normal glucose processing is impaired. If these stages are disrupted, then there will be an impact on hormonal release.

Sleep and Jet Lag

You don't have to change your daily activity pattern very much to experience the impact on the digestive system. I mean, who hasn't gone on a business trip or family vacation to only suffer later from all the rich food, alcohol, and crazy schedule, all played out in another time zone?

Historically, travel across time zones didn't really matter much when using ship, train, or automobile, but the impact of jet lag really became an issue with the development of air travel. While it was known among military personnel, who were the first to learn about "jet-lag," the advent of commercial air travel brought this experience to the masses.

The investigation of circadian cycles in hibernating animals was quite evolved by the time jet lag began to impact people. This early work showed that cells within brain structures (e.g., hypothalamus and the suprachiasmic nucleus) were important in the control of normal sleep-wake cycles. Also, outside stimuli, called *Zeitgebers,* are instrumental in maintaining or changing this pattern (23). The most important of these *Zeitgebers* is light which entrains our system to the 24-hour cycle of the Earth.

Dr. Charles Ehret was director of the Division of Biological and Medical Research group at the Argonne National Laboratory in Illinois, one of the many labs that evolved from the Manhattan Project. While primarily a zoologist, Dr. Ehret became a leader in the newly evolving field of chronobiology after a brief time investigating the impact of electromagnetic energy on cells. His work on the eukaryotic circadian clock was developed during the 1960's and early 1970's, which lead him to the idea of how to synchronize an individual to a time zone during jet travel (24). He believed the solution for countering jet lag was to alter metabolism through energy substrates (high protein or high carbohydrates) a few days before leaving. This substrate change acted as *Zeitgebers* to reset the biological drive for energy and, eventually, sleep. The diet was reviewed (25) by the *New York Times* nutrition editor, Jane Brody, in 1983 with great fanfare, but even that didn't convince people that the answer to their jet lag was as simple as changing their diet.

A study published in *Military Medicine* (26) reported that National Guard troops who did not practice the Argonne diet before deployment to Korea were 7.5% more likely to experience jet lag than those who used the diet. In addition, the authors noted that physical activity seemed to be an important factor for preventing jet-lag. Although this was from a small, select study, the data does show that in certain populations limited improvements in combating jet lag can be obtained through nutritional and food schedule interventions as proposed by Dr. Ehret.

It is interesting that Dr. Ehret used the basic nutritional components of carbohydrates and protein to phase shift the body. Whether he and his group knew it or not, they were in fact, altering the gut microbiota which have since proven to be instrumental in the mammalian digestive process. In fact, there are reports that these gut microbes have an evolutionary cycle of their own (27).

Sleep and Gut Microbiota

How this all relates to sleep disruption and obesity is perhaps summed up in a very creative study done by Christopher Thais and colleagues (28) from the Department of Immunology, Weizmann Institute of Science, in Israel. From previous research, the authors noted that intestinal gut microbiota exhibited diurnal oscillations and that feeding altered the microbiotic composition and rhythmicity of the host organism (e.g., mice). Thais and colleagues showed that gut oscillations could be altered by transplanting gut fecal material from normal, non-mutated mice into a genetic variation that lacked gut oscillations. It was noted that after transplantation, these genetically altered mice eventually developed gut microbiotic oscillations that were similar to the wild-type mouse. This experiment demonstrated that the gut oscillations could, indeed, be controlled by contents within the intestines. Then, the authors examined the influence of gut microbiota on time-shifted (jet lagged) and normal control mice given a high-fat diet. The jet lagged mice eventually exhibited weight gain and impaired glucose intolerance within six weeks of exposure to the time change. What this all means is that there is a lot more going on in your digestive system than you ever imagined. Subtle changes in your circadian clock can induce very significant alternations in your metabolism, leading to potential weight gain and diabetes.

37

Sleep and Metabolic Syndrome

Metabolic syndrome is a disease condition related to a large number of physiological, biochemical, and hormonal imbalances. While not a new term, the understanding and conceptualization of the term "metabolic syndrome" played out over a period of 250 years beginning with Morgagni in the mid-18th Century and ending with Reaven in 1988 (29). The impact of metabolic syndrome can be seen from an International Diabetes Federation (IDF) report, "It is estimated that around 20-25 per cent of the world's adult population have the metabolic syndrome and they are twice as likely to die from and three times as likely to have a heart attack or stroke compared with people without the syndrome. In addition, people with metabolic syndrome have a fivefold greater risk of developing type 2 diabetes." The most current definition of metabolic syndrome was published by the International Diabetes Federation in 2006 (30) and shown below:

According to the new IDF definition, for a person to be defined as having the metabolic syndrome they must have central obesity (defined as waist circumference $\geq$ 94cm for Europid men and $\geq$ 80cm for Europid women) plus any two of the following four factors:

- raised triglyceride (TG) level: $\geq$ 150 mg/dL (1.7 mmol/L), or specific treatment for this lipid abnormality
- reduced HDL cholesterol: < 40 mg/dL (1.03 mmol/L*) in males and < 50 mg/dL (1.29 mmol/L*) in females, or specific treatment for this lipid abnormality
- raised blood pressure (BP): systolic BP $\geq$ 130 or diastolic BP $\geq$ 85 mm Hg, or treatment of previously diagnosed hypertension
- raised fasting plasma glucose (FPG): $\geq$ 100 mg/dL (5.6 mmol/L), or previously diagnosed type 2 diabetes.

The importance of "central obesity" cannot be underscored in terms of the development of metabolic syndrome. There is accumulating data which shows that fat stores from the central or deep fat elicit much greater danger than fat that accumulates under the skin (31). It follows the "apple versus pear" analogy that you may remember from decades past (32).

How does sleep or the lack of sleep impact metabolic syndrome and associated diabetes?

There is perhaps no better research data to answer this question than that from the laboratory of Dr. Kari Knutson and colleagues out of the University of Chicago. Knutson and colleagues have elucidated many of the physiological systems impacted by poor sleep (33). The majority of their research has focused on the impact of sleep disturbance on glucose metabolism leading to diabetes and obesity, which are linked with metabolic syndrome. Knutson states in the *American Journal of Human Biology (34)* that "given the potential link between inadequate sleep and obesity, a critical next step is to identify the social, cultural and environmental determinants of sleep, which would help to identify vulnerable populations." The figure below, is taken from this review paper, and shows the impact of inadequate sleep on the many processes within the body.

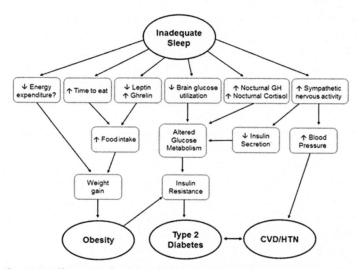

Figure reprinted by permission from Wiley and published in the American J Human Biology (2006) 24(3): 361-371. Schematic representation of possible mechanistic pathways linking inadequate sleep to obesity, diabetes, cardiovascular disease (CVD), and hypertension (HTN), GH – growth hormone.

39

Short sleep duration in children and adults has been reported to increase the incidence of weight gain and obesity (35). From the Wisconsin Sleep Cohort Study, it was reported that sleeping five hours versus the eight hour baseline increased body weight by 4% to 5% showing that small disturbances in normal sleep can lead to dramatic effects (36). Moreover, there are associated studies which show an increased likelihood of obesity and diabetes with alterations in sleep duration, sleep cycle, and quality of sleep. Much of these all report some relationship between glucose regulation and circadian rhythmicity, similar to what was proposed by Dr. Ehret from his work on eukaryotic cells. It seems apparent then that maintaining consistent sleep habits are one of the key critical elements to maintaining good health.

Sleep and Food Selection

I am sure we have all experienced the impact of poor sleep on our daily lives—whether helping the kids get ready for school, preparing for a business meeting, or trying to focus on a particular task—things just don't go smoothly. There are three areas that can be attributed to the slow progression of weight gain: lack of physical activity, poor nutritional choices, and inconsistent eating patterns. The figure below shows how poor sleep leads to low energy and focus, resulting in a lack of interest in physical activity, leading to a low energy state.

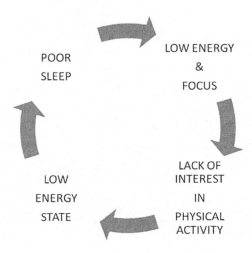

Now couple the process above with the impact of low sleep on our conscious or sub-conscious decisions. Here, poor sleep reduces the ability to make good choices, often resulting in increased eating and food binging, and even poor or inadequate food selection.

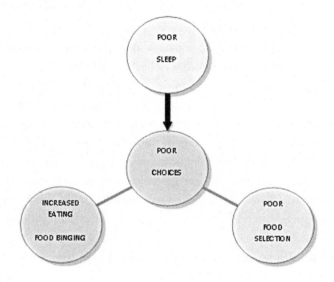

We wake up from a bad night's sleep wanting to exercise but too tired to carry out the task. We then gravitate to poor food choices by selecting that yummy pastry or two. Now, compound that process over an extended period of time, and that slow, progressive weight gain begins. To break this cycle requires tremendous effort and will. This is where the use of peer pressure or group exercise comes into play. Let others pull you along in their wake as they exercise. Soon, you will be the one pulling along others toward a healthy lifestyle and living.

Do you come home from work after a long day and just grab some kind of food? Well, don't despair because there is new data suggesting that selection process or ethical behavior is often impacted when made during an individual's period of sleep deprivation and low energy (37). There are a couple of mechanisms for this selection process.

One is the low energy state which drives the desire for carbohydrate rich foods. Dr. Judith Wurtman at the Massachusetts Institute of Technology (MIT) coined the term "carbohydrate cravers" from her research on student food selection (38). Her collaborative research concluded that when confronted with a choice, most people sought out sugary carbohydrate foods, rather than protein or fat based foods. This work was criticized at some level due to the hedonistic or decadent appearance of carbohydrate-rich foods like a donut compared to that of beef jerky or butter. It was felt that the visual image had much more to do with the selection than any neurological or biochemical tendency to the substrate itself. However, the findings of this early work was recently supported through a selection process of beverage drink containing the different ingredients. Corsica and Spring (39) reported that carbohydrate cravers felt an improved mood after ingesting a carbohydrate-rich beverage versus that of a high-protein beverage. In addition, Stice and colleagues reported that sugar, more than fat or protein, effectively activates reward regions within the brain (40).

The second component of poor food selection may come from the neural network not related to energy balance at all. Chapman and colleagues investigated food purchase behavior in 14 men who were tasked with making food purchases at a supermarket after a night of eight hours of sleep versus a night with no sleep (41). The treatments were separated by four weeks to prevent any habituation, and subjects were given one day to acclimate to the experimental setting before each intervention. After the sleep deprivation night, the subjects purchased more calories and grams of food when compared to the normal baseline sleep night. How this plays out in reality is hard to say, but it does show that our choices can be manipulated through sleep disruption. Perhaps a good idea is to make important decisions, whether about food or finances, after a good night's sleep and a full belly.

Food Availability and Weight Gain

There is new research out of the Salk Institute suggesting that weight loss can be managed better if a person eats within a 12-hour window and then fasts for the remaining 12 hours (42). Well, don't we do that already in our normal schedule? Do you really get up in the middle of the night and consume food?

While the research conducted at the Salk Institute is thorough and descriptive, it may have limitations when applied to human application. For the most part, their work is done exclusively on mice, which represents a slightly different metabolic profile. For instance, they mention the involvement of brown fat in their metabolic cycle, which unfortunately, is not abundant in humans. However, it makes intuitive sense that the more you limit the hours of available food consumption, the less food you will consume. But, does it?

Hatori and colleagues (43) showed that by limiting access to food, mice had lower amounts of body fat when compared to mice that could eat at their liberty or *ad libitum*. If the mice were allowed to have longer periods from which to graze from the eating trough, there was an associated increase in body fat stores. The authors provided a tremendous amount of data regarding different metabolic pathways and energy distribution that all revolve around our good friends: sugar and insulin. As stated in their discussion, the reduced availability of insulin limits its ability to store energy as fat, and the lack of insulin while fasting increases the drive to burn fat. Basically, be measured in your eating at all times to reduce excess caloric intake and use fasting to help drive your metabolic engine to burn body fat.

These studies suggest that when one limits the window for food consumption, there is a beneficial effect on the circadian clock and metabolic regulators. The significant increases in gene expression of lipid enzymes, result in greater fat utilization and less fat storage in the liver. This is very important because one off-shoot of obesity is non-alcohol fatty liver disease (NAFLD). This condition is increasingly becoming a concern around the world because of its profound impact on mortality (44).

In closing, the essence of this chapter is that one must look at the many aspects of life, in this case sleep, to help understand and change behavior or outcomes regarding health. You should consider sleep as an integral part of your weight management program. Take the time to consider how your sleep patterns may play a role in your health and body weight challenges. You may find that just a little more sleep, may go a long way toward better living and longevity.

Simple things you can do:

- Determine what sleep schedule works best for you.
- Set boundaries with roommates and family about sleep schedules.
- Avoid sleep antagonists at least three hours before bed.
- Set up your bedroom to be sleep friendly; take out the TV, computer.
- Eliminate tablet and mobile phone use before bed.
- Use relaxation techniques to help quiet your mind and body before bed.

Cited References

1. Cohen, E. (2011, June 23). Does life online give you popcorn brain? CNN. Retrieved from http://www.cnn.com/2011/HEALTH/06/23/tech.popcorn.brain.ep/

2. Nohara, K., Yoo, S. H., & Chen, Z. J. (2015). Manipulating the circadian and sleep cycles to protect against metabolic disease. Frontiers in Endocrinology (Lausanne), 6(35). doi:10.3389/fendo.2015.00035

3. Vriend, J., & Reiter, R. J. (2015). Melatonin feedback on clock genes: a theory involving the proteasome. Journal of Pineal Research, 58(1), 1-11.

4. Porkka-Heiskanen, T., Alanko, L., Kalinchuk, A. & Stenberg, D. (2002). Adenosine and sleep. Sleep Medicine Reviews, 6, 321-332. doi:10.1053/smrv.2001.0201

5. Riberio, J. A. & Sebastião, A. M. (2010). Caffeine and adenosine. Journal of Alzheimer's Disease, 20, S3-S15.

6. Schwartz, J. R., & Roth, T. (2008). Neurophysiology of sleep and wakefulness: basic science and clinical implications. Current Neuropharmacology, 6(4), 367–378.

7. Shambroom, J. R., Fábregras, S. E. & Johnstone, J. (2012). Validation of an automated wireless system to monitor sleep in healthy adults. Journal of Sleep Research, 21, 221-230.

8. Tonetti, L., Cellini, N., de Zambotti, M., Fabbri, M., Martoni, M., Fábregras, S. E., Stegagno, L. & Natale, V. (2013). Polysomnographic validation of a wireless dry headband technology for sleep monitoring in healthy young adults. Physiology Behavior, 118, 185-188.

9. Technology Quarterly. (2012, March), Counting every moment. The Economist.

10. Kryger, M. H., Roth, T., Dement, W. C. (Eds). (2000). Principles and practices of sleep medicine (3rd ed). Philadelphia: W. B. Saunders Company.

11. Colten, H. R., Altevogt, B. M. (Eds). (2006). Sleep disorders and sleep deprivation: an unmet public health problem. Institute of Medicine (US) Committee on Sleep Medicine and Research, Washington, DC: National Academies Press. Retrieved from http://www.ncbi.nlm.nih.gov/books/NBK19960/

12. Bonnet, M. H. & Arand, D. L. (2003). Clinical effects of sleep fragmentation versus sleep deprivation. Sleep Medicine Reviews, 7, 297-310.

13. Bonnet, M. H. (1987). Sleep restoration as a function of periodic awakening, movement, or electroencephalographic change. Sleep, 10, 364-373.

14. Morrison, A. (2011). The discovery of REM sleep: the death knell of the passive theory of sleep. In B. N. Mallick, S. R. Pandi-Perumal, R. W. McCarley, & A. R. Morrison (Eds.) Rapid eye movement sleep: regulation and function. Cambridge: Cambridge University Press.

15. Morselli, L., Leproult, R., Balbo, M. & Spiegal, K. (2010). Role of sleep duration in the regulation of glucose metabolism and appetite. Best Practice & Research Clinical Endocrinology & Metabolism, 24, 687-702.

16. Taheri, S. (2007). Sleep and metabolism: bringing pieces of the jigsaw together. Sleep Medicine Reviews, 11, 159-162.

17. Smith, A. G., & Muscat, G. E. (2005). Skeletal muscle and nuclear hormone receptors: implications for cardiovascular and metabolic disease. International Journal of Biochemical & Cell Biology, 37(10), 2047-2063.

18. Aronoff, S. L., Berkowitz, K., Shreiner, B., & Want, L. (2004). Glucose metabolism and regulation: beyond insulin and glucagon. Diabetes Spectrum, 3, 183-190.

19. Sanz, C., Gautier, J. F., & Hanaire, H. (2010). Physical exercise for the prevention and treatment of type 2 diabetes. Diabetes Metabolism, 36(5), 346-351.

20. Mesarwi, O., Polak, J., Jun, J. & Polotsky, V. Y. (2013). Sleep disorders and the development of insulin resistance and obesity. Endocrinology and metabolism Clinics of North America, 42, 617-634.

21. Kalsbeek, A., la Fleur, S., & Fliers, E. (2014). Circadian control of glucose metabolism. Molecular Metabolism, 3(4), 372-383.

22. Roenneberg, T., & Merrow, M. (2007). Entrainment of the human circadian clock. Cold Spring Harbor Symposium Quantitative Biology, 72, 293-299.

23. Tahara, Y., & Shibata, S. (2013). Chronobiology and nutrition. Neuroscience, 253, 78-88. doi: 10.1016/j.neuroscience.2013.08.049

24. Ehret, C. F., & Scanlon, L. W. (1997). Overcoming jet lag. New York, NY: Berkeley Trade.

25. Brody, J. E. (1983). The jet lag diet. New York, NY: The New York Times.

26. Reynolds, N. C., & Montgomery, R. (2002). Using the Argonne Diet in jet lag prevention: deployment of troops across nine time zones. Military Medicine, 167(6): 451-53.

27. Quercia, S., Candela, M., Giuliani, C., Turroni, S., Luiselli, D., Rampelli, S., Brigidi, P., Franceschi, C., Bacalini, M. G., Garagnani, P., Pirazzini, C. (2014). From lifetime to evolution: timescales of human gut microbiota adaptation. Frontiers of Microbiology, 4(5), 587.

28. Thaiss, C. A., Zeevi, D., Levy, M., Zilberman-Schapira, G., Suez, J., Tengeler, A. C.,...Elinav, E. (2014). Transkingdom control of microbiota diurnal oscillations promotes metabolic homeostasis. Cell, 159, 514-529.

29. Crepaldi, G., & Maggi, S. (2006). The metabolic syndrome: a historical context [Special Issue]. Diabetes Voice, 51. Retrieved from http://www.idf.org/sites/default/files/attachments/issue_43_en.pdf

30. International Diabetes Federation. Definition of metabolic syndrome. Retrieved from http://www.idf.org/metabolic-syndrome

31. Philipsen, A., Jørgensen, M. E., Vistisen, D., Sandbaek, A., Almdal, T. P., Christiansen, J. S., Lauritzen, T., & Witte, D. R. (2015). Associations between ultrasound measures of abdominal fat distribution and indices of glucose metabolism in a population at high risk of type 2 diabetes: the ADDITION-PRO study. PLoS One, 10(4).

32. Rimm, A. A, Hartz, A. J., & Fischer, M. E. (1988). A weight shape index for assessing risk of disease in 44,820 women. Journal of Clinical Epidemiology, 41(5), 459-465.

33. Knutson, K. L., Spiegel, K., Penev, P. & Cauter, E. V. (2007). The metabolic consequences of sleep deprivation. Sleep Medicine Reviews, 11, 163-178.

34. Knutson, K. L. (2012). Does inadequate sleep play a role in vulnerability to obesity? American Journal of Human Biology, 24, 361-371.

35. Morselli, L. L., Knutson, K. L., & Mokhlesi, B. (2012). Sleep and insulin resistance in adolescents. Sleep, 35(10), 1313-1314.

36. Magee, L. & Hale, L. (2012). Longitudinal associations between sleep duration and subsequent weight gain: a systematic review. Sleep Medicine Reviews, 16, 231-241.

37. Anderson, C., & Dickinson, D. L. (2010). Bargaining and trust: the effects of 36-h total sleep deprivation on socially interactive decisions. Journal of Sleep Research, 19(1), 54-63.

38. Wurtman, J. J. (1988). Carbohydrate cravings: a disorder of food intake and mood. Clinical Neuropharmacology, 11(S1), S139-145.

39. Corsica, J. A, & Spring, B. J. (2008). Carbohydrate craving: a double-blind, placebo-controlled test of the self-medication hypothesis. Eating Behaviors, 9(4), 447-454.

40. Stice, E., Burger, K., & Yokum, S. (2013). Relative ability of fat and sugar tastes to activate reward, gustatory and somatosensory regions. American Journal of Clinical Nutrition, 98, 1377-1384.

41. Chapman, C. D., Nilsson, E. K., Nilsson, V. C., Cedernaes, J., Rangtell, F. H., Vogel, H., Benedict, C. (2013). Acute sleep deprivation increases food purchasing in men. Obesity, 21, 555-560.

42. Chaix, A., Zarrinpar, A, & Panda, S. (2014). Time-restricted feeding is a preventative and therapeutic intervention against diverse nutritional challenges. Cell Metabolism, 20, 991-1005.

43. Hatori, M., Vollmers, C., Zarrinpar, A., DiTacchio, L., Bushong, E. A., Gill, S.,…Panda, S. (2012). Time restricted feeding without reducing caloric intake prevents metabolic diseases in mice fed a high fat diet. Cell Metabolism, 15, 848-860.

44. Haufe, S., Haas, V., Utz, W., Birkenfeld, A. L., et al. (2013). Long-lasting improvements in liver fat and metabolism despite body weight regain after dietary weight loss. Diabetes Care, 36(11), 3786-3792.

Additional Resources

Bonnet, M. H. & Arand, D. L. (1996). Metabolic rate and the restorative function of sleep. *Physiology Behavior, 59,* 777-782.

Hale, L. & Berger, L. M. (2011). Sleep duration and childhood obesity: moving from research to practice. *SLEEP, 34,* 1153-1154.

Haslam, D. R. & Abraham, P. (1987). Sleep loss and military performance. In G. Belenky (Ed.), *contemporary studies in combat psychiatry* (pp. 167-184). Westport, CT: Greenwood Press.

Horne, J. A. (1988). *Why we sleep: the functions of sleep in humans and other mammals* (pp. 12-75). Oxford: Oxford University Press.

Kouchaki, M. & Smith, I. H. (2014). The morning morality effect. *Psychological Science, 25,* 95-102.

Magee, L. & Hale, L. (2012). Longitudinal associations between sleep duration and subsequent weight gain: a systematic review. *Sleep Medicine Reviews, 16,* 231-241.

Punjabi, N. E., Shahar, E., Redline, S., Gottlieb, D. J., Givelber, R. & Resnick, H. E. (2004). Sleep- disordered breathing, glucose intolerance, and insulin resistance. *American Journal of Epidemiology, 160,* 521-530.

Reaven, G. M. (1988). Banting lecture: role of insulin resistance in human disease. *Diabetes, 37*(12), 1595-1607

Sato, M., Murakami, M., Node, K., Matsumura, R. & Akashi, M. (2014). The role of the endocrine system in feeding-induced tissue-specific circadian entrainment. *Cell, 8,* 393-401.

3
Slow Down

The circadian nature of the planet, and the physiological processes needed to support and maintain the human body weren't made for a 24/7 lifestyle (1). I mean, when the sun set in your great grandparent's day, there wasn't a heck of a lot to do. They went to bed, had a good night's sleep, and then woke up the next day, at first light. They had a solid breakfast, went about their day burning calories out on the farm or ranch, and came home as the sun set.

It was simpler then, and you need to get "simple" back into your life now. It is the technology that makes it so darned easy to be plugged in all the time, but you are in control—so un-plug now!

Depending on your age, you may remember when times were a little slower—when "instant access" meant days or weeks, not seconds. You had to wait for a letter to be received, read, and then returned. Or…when you had to wait until you got to your home or office to use the landline to make a telephone call. Then, you hoped that the person you were calling was home to answer; otherwise, you had to leave a message (given they had an answering machine) and wait for them to return your call. Phew! I am exhausted just thinking about how cumbersome that process was back then. My, how things have changed!

The realization that our fast-paced world has had a dramatic impact on people came to me when I was traveling a lot for work. I was on the go at home and at work, always moving and traveling. I started to notice that I was aging quicker and gaining weight more than I liked. As I started to focus inward on my own aging process, I started to look around at my friends, colleagues, and fellow travelers, who seemed to be showing similar aging processes—fatigue, wrinkles, poor posture, and weight gain.

The full impact of such a lifestyle came full circle when I started watching a neighborhood friend begin a new career. His prior employment kept him at one location with normal hours, but as he began to travel, I noticed a change. He started to age before my eyes—his once coal black hair turned to salt and pepper, and his eyes had that tired, sad look. His skin had a dull pallor and his middle started to expand. At that point I knew I had to slow down, and I knew I had to write this book.

When I began writing this book, I soon learned that there wasn't a heck of a lot of research on "slowing down." The closest information that I could find usually dealt with yoga or meditation. When you think about it, how do you *measure* slowing down? What are the important metrics to use? Is slowing down the same for everyone?

We are learning, each and every day, about the main organ that controls us all—the brain. We are learning that the brain and its network of neurons and connections need a chance to re-boot and refresh (2). The brain needs time to sort through tragedy, drama, information, happiness, and sorrow. The brain needs to coordinate stuff we learned, and forget stuff we don't need to remember. Our body organs (e.g., liver, kidney, heart) need to regenerate energy stores and cleanse themselves of metabolic byproducts.

By participating in meditation or yoga, one must slowdown in order to focus and perform the activity. In our fast-paced world, the acceptance of slowing down or the ability to slow down is not common. How many people do you know that are constantly challenged by not having enough time to complete their tasks at work and at home? How many times during the day and/or week do you wish you had more time to do what is asked of you—by your boss, your spouse, and your kids?

Shift Work, Not So Good

Today, we still function on a 9 to 5 employment schedule. We sit in our cubicles of some kind, and do what we are told. We are told that if you need to exercise, do it before or after work. If you need to go to the doctor or go to the cleaners, go after work. If you need a "mental health" day, sneak a vacation day. This kind of attitude does not bode well for someone needing a slower pace in hopes of better health. There are signs all around about how this fast pace can cause health issues. I will address two groups that perhaps typify this problem—nurses and police officers.

Have you ever noticed during your annual physical exam that the healthcare staff look a little tired and overweight? Ever visit a family member in the hospital and notice that most of the nursing staff are overworked and overweight? How about that college friend who always wanted a career in law enforcement? Out of the police academy, they were solid as a rock, but over the years they've gotten a little soft around the middle.

It's not them, it's the shift work and long hours. Intuitively, it seems that a person can be more efficient working a 10- or 12-hour shift rather than 8 hours. When you consider the wind up and wind down time of an 8-hour day, real work time is perhaps only 6 hours. However, there is increasing research showing that long work days (greater than 12 hours) and shift work (evening and graveyard) cause significant health problems.

53

A recent report by Rachel Craig and colleagues (3) from the Health and Social Care Information Centre out of the United Kingdom presents very compelling data about the impact of shift work outside of the normal 7 AM to 7 PM work schedule. Some of the major findings include:

- Shift workers were more likely than non-shift workers to be obese.
- Men and women in shift work were more likely than non-shift workers to have diabetes (10% of both men and women in shift work, compared with 9% and 7% respectively of those not working shifts).
- Daily fruit and vegetable consumption was lower among shift workers than non-shift workers.

The impact of shift work on health outcomes has been reported in a variety of occupations and across countries. Claire Caruso reviewed the negative impact of shiftwork and long work hours in U.S. nurses (4). This thoughtful and comprehensive review outlined the impact of shift work on sleep, neurocognitive function and performance, worker injury and error, and poor health behaviors. The effect on these U.S.-based nurses was similar to that found in nurses at eighteen public Brazilian hospitals. Griep and colleagues (5) reported that the number of years worked at night increased body mass index significantly for both men and women. Also, Jang and colleagues reported that Korean adult workers performing manual labor greater than 60 hours per week showed greater risk for obesity (6).

The reason for such an impact of shift work relates as much to the available sleep hours, as it does to the actual time of work. It is intuitive that the longer work day means less time available for non-work and sleep activity. This is especially true for those individuals serving as caregivers for children and/or parents. Interestingly, being out of work or unemployed led to less weight gain and more weight loss than when employed (7). This was the finding from the Australian Longitudinal Study of Women's Health on over 9276 women aged 45-50 years at baseline. The authors concluded that as women work longer hours, they were more likely to make lifestyle choices that were associated with weight gain—less physical activity, poor dietary practices and personal choices, to name a few.

If one can manage to get enough sleep, and manage to work better, what can one do to slow down? In reality, there are any number of ways to slow down. Some people read, others do puzzles, others watch television, and some just want silence for contemplation. I find that people often forget about this activity. In a world where we are bombarded constantly by noise, I find silence to be very therapeutic and productive.

Meditation, Yoga, and Mindfulness

In looking through the scientific and medical literature, the most common activities associated with slowing down are meditation and yoga. There is a new movement that has become quite popular. The term that I am speaking of is "mindfulness" or being mindful of one's surroundings. Another way to think of it is "being in the moment, aware of your surroundings, your breath, your heartbeat and your presence."

Go ahead and try it! If you need some help, follow these steps:

1. Close your eyes, but open your ears.
2. Hear yourself breathing; hear and feel your heartbeat.
3. Put your mind at peace, thinking only about this moment in time.
4. Now, stay here until you are ready to come back to reality.

It may take some practice to do it without thinking about your work, your kids, or social media accounts.

The exercise above is the essence of "slowing down." In our fast-paced world, it is very hard to achieve, so we often need help or guidance. The more you do, the more you learn. Don't expect that you will be able to achieve a sense of peace immediately. It takes time, so use it to your benefit.

Mindful Living

I think it is pretty clear that most of us eat because of emotional stress, and many times this carries over to our sleep. There is some recent research showing that the use of mindful-based, behavioral intervention has some impact on sleep and eating disorders. Corsica and colleagues (8) looked at mindful-based stress reduction techniques on stress-eating and the risk of obesity. After six weeks, overweight participants were better able to reduce their stress level and stress eating. This was supported by the work of Dalen and colleagues who looked at participants recruited from the YMCA (9). The participants followed a curriculum called Mindful Eating and Living (MEAL) which included training in mindfulness meditation, mindful eating, and group discussion. After six weeks, the ten obese patients demonstrated improved control in stress-eating, binge eating, depression, and experienced a significant loss in body weight.

Even the U.S. Marine Corps uses mindful-based techniques in helping their warriors cope with the stress of deployment. In a recent paper published in the *American Journal of Psychiatry* (10), Marine infantry platoons preparing for combat exercises were divided into two groups. One group received the usual training routine and the other received education on mindful-based mind fitness training (MMFT) emphasizing inner physiological awareness, attentional control, and tolerance of present-moment experiences. The authors concluded that those Marines experienced with MMFT, performed better and adapted better to the stressful stimuli than those who did not have experience. Moreover, having had prior MMFT experience led to quicker recovery times.

While the term "mindful" might be a new concept, the power of the mind has been known for centuries. A book from the 1920's taught children about hard work and optimism through the exploits of a "little engine that could." Norman Vincent Peale championed this concept in his book (11), *The Power of Positive Thinking*, first published in 1952. The power of his message directed many individuals to pursue challenges beyond their imaginations. We have come to learn so much more about the brain since then, but in reality, what we know today is only a fraction of what is to be learned. So be mindful, you might just get a little more benefit than just slowing down!

In fact, there are a couple of interesting studies showing how meditation can reduce brain tissue loss with age and help older people sleep better. As reported in the *Frontiers of Psychology* (12), Luders and colleagues presented data showing that people who had meditated for 20 years or longer, tended to have higher brain volume than age-matched controls. This was significant because it is known that brain size, vasculature, and cognition change negatively with age (13). Fjell and colleagues (14) conducted an evaluation of 132 healthy, elderly (60 – 91 years of age) patients unlikely to develop Alzheimer's disease (AD). Using magnetic resonance imaging (MRI), the authors found that over a one-year period, healthy individuals experienced reductions in most areas of the brain, suggesting that not all changes with age reflect a risk for dementia. While changes in brain volume cannot be predictive of AD, activities that maintain or increase brain activity or structure are important for high cognitive function with aging (15).

Ask an older family member or friend about their sleep habits, and you will surely get an earful. Poor sleep seems to be a hallmark of aging with a variety of known and unknown causes (16). However, a recent study out of the University of Southern California showed that participating in a six week sleep hygiene and education program improved response on a sleep quality questionnaire (17). The subjects had the benefit of a certified mindfulness and meditation counselor, who taught them how to make their bedrooms more conducive to sleep, and learn how to relax and decrease physiological arousal, that often leads to poor sleep and insomnia.

Mindfulness seems to have caught on not only at home but also at work. There have been several articles in business journals and social media about the use of mindfulness to help engage and improve employee performance. However, Dr. David Brendel, an executive coach and counselor, worries that "mindfulness" has become so over-used that it may lead to a backlash against those that practice and endorse its value (18). He says that many individuals use the concept of "mindfulness" to opt out of making critical decisions. In some cases, managers become so engaged with the concept that they force it upon others. These issues are counter to what one should gain from "mindfulness" practice and underscore the importance of self-selection and balance.

One can also think of "mindful" in terms of meditation, and meditation often leads one to think of yoga. This activity has been around for centuries and is most often associated with Hindi or Ayurvedic healing. It can be slow and passive or fast and active. It works to stretch and relax the muscles, as much as it does to strengthen them. If you have ever experienced a good yoga session, you know what I am talking about. If you haven't done it, give it a try. Challenge yourself, and be amazed.

Yoga and Health

Over the years there have been many attempts to quantify and clarify the benefits of yoga on health outcomes. Yoga is not just one thing; it is a collection of activities that encompasses a number of variables and interactions. Naturally, this complexity makes it hard to show benefit, but there has been an increasing attempt to document the benefit(s) of yoga.

While I could discuss any number of newer studies on yoga therapy, I have chosen three which show the value of participating in such an activity. In 2012, Yadav and colleagues published a preliminary trial in the *Journal of Alternative and Complementary Medicine* (19). In this small, non-randomized study, overweight and obese patients, with chronic inflammatory diseases, participated in yoga therapy for 10 days. The main findings were reductions in stress markers for those suffering from chronic inflammation. In 2013, Rioux and Ritenbaugh, performed a retrospective review of clinical trials using yoga as an intervention for weight loss (20). The investigators evaluated each study based on duration, frequency of yoga practice, intensity of each practice, number of yoga activities or elements, inclusion of dietary modification, inclusion of a residential component, number of weight-related outcome measures, and discussion of yogic elements. The authors concluded that therapeutic yoga programs are frequently effective for promoting weight loss and improving body composition. Finally, Manchanda and Madan published a paper in 2014 in *Clinical Research Cardiology* (21). They concluded from their review of published yoga and meditation research that participation was beneficial for primary and secondary prevention of cardiovascular disease.

Take a Sabbatical

Another benefit of slowing down may be that you actually enjoy the activities that you do. There have been a few studies showing that those people who take time to step away from the job, tend to have a more energized feeling, and actually think better of their work than those who are consumed with work 24/7. The intent of the academic sabbatical was to allow the professor an opportunity for self-improvement, which hopefully would then come back to benefit the university and the students. And, some companies have provided something similar to their senior staff needing a break from the stress of daily management. In both of these cases, the individual is usually provided some kind of compensation to help cover expenses. Naturally, this is the best case scenario, regardless of the amount of support. While not quite the same, a couple of mental health days, might be just as good.

What if you can't get a year sabbatical or even a mental health day? How about if you can't get your boss to reduce your work week from 60 hours to 40 hours? Or, to switch from a 12 hour to an 8 hour per day shift? Well, don't despair. There is an answer that just might help you be more productive and live longer.

Go Ahead, Take a Nap

Of course, I am talking about a *siesta* or an afternoon nap. We know that the "siesta" has been part of Spanish tradition for centuries. It harkens back to the days of Spanish glory and the need to allow the peasants a little respite from the afternoon Mediterranean heat. This break allowed the workers to be more productive in the fields and later, factories. The main component of a siesta is the 20- to 40-minute nap that allows the workers to re-energize. However, the industrialized economies soon realized that this schedule did not allow them to maximize their productivity. Ultimately, the siesta has become extinct in most non-Spanish based economies.

It is not that the allure of a short nap disappeared from society. It just became something that one didn't mention with much pride or honesty. Who hasn't had the thought of a good nap after lunch or that late afternoon meeting? As we discussed in Chapter 2, the drive for sleep is strong, just like the drive to eat, and it takes quite a bit of discipline to counter these urges. However, for some odd reason, we are a little better suited at preventing that nap. Caffeine was an early stimulant, and remains to this day to be the energizer of choice. Sadly, along came those energy drink boosters filled with caffeine and sugar, perhaps helping to fight fatigue but also possibly contributing to diabetes and obesity.

There was a time when people bragged about pulling all-nighters or pushing through an 18 hour shift writing code or working a double at the factory. Or, those young medical interns serving their time on the 36-hour shift covering the emergency room. But, somewhere along the way, people started to question whether this was such a good idea. Not surprisingly, one of the first groups to investigate the impact of sleep on performance, was the military. Dr. Belenky and his colleagues from the U.S. Army Walter Reed Medical Center were pioneers in the use of newer technology on measuring performance as a function of sleep deprivation (22). This group expanded our knowledge on sleep cycles and pharmacological intervention (23).

I talked earlier about the effect of shift work on nurses and law enforcement personnel. Longer days and off-cycle work schedules were reported as important factors contributing to health issues and human error. In reviewing the literature, I came across numerous recent studies looking at the impact of naps on alertness and performance. Sallinen and colleagues reported in 1998, that naps less than one hour, seemed to improve alertness for individuals working a night shift (24). The nap allowed the workers to respond to visual signals better during the second half of their night shift.

Smith-Coggins and colleagues concluded that by taking a nap at 3 AM, study participants were better able to perform later on tasks related to vigilance, memory recall, and fine motor skills, when compared to no-nap controls (24). Furthermore, Schweitzer and colleagues reported that naps plus caffeine improved psychomotor vigilance and alertness in a group of night shift workers (26).

While a nap may normally be considered an afternoon event, it is quite evident from research that a nap can be quite powerful when taken at any time of day or night, given the work schedule. In keeping with their goal to improve and enhance performance during battle, the military continues to investigate the impact of sleep on solider performance. The U.S. Army Military Medicine division has published the "Performance Leaders Guide" which covers the main concepts in their more comprehensive *Performance Triad: Activity, Nutrition and Sleep.* The 12-page guide is short, concise, and to the point (27). For a more extensive review on the topic of human performance, I highly recommend the book by Hancock and Szalma, *Performance Under Stress* (28). The book is filled with excellent chapters written by the leading experts in the field of military ergonomics, sports performance, and environmental physiology.

While there have been many other scientists and clinicians investigating sleep over the past few decades, there are only a few that have looked at naps. Dr. Sara Mednick, from the University of California at Riverside, is such a person. She has spent her career investigating the impact of sleep on cognitive function and performance. In fact, as she says in her book, *Take a Nap, Change Your Life*, it was the short naps on a "ratty old couch" in the lab of Harvard University's Psychology department that launched her interest in the field (29).

Dr. Mednick believes that people can't function at optimum levels, unless they take a nap to restore mental energy and function. Not surprisingly, her research has shown that naps need to be taken within a specific time window. This relates to the circadian nature of our physiological and hormonal systems that we have discussed repeatedly throughout this book. From her research she developed the "Nap Wheel" which allows an individual to customize their nap schedule. How cool is that?

In closing, the timing of when you should "slow down" is now! How each person "slows down" will vary, but it should be done sooner rather than later. Some people might be able to do it cold turkey while others may need to ease into it. However it is done, I will say that it will be one of the most rewarding moments in your life. You will be faced with putting a higher value on time, instead of material things.

Simple things you can do:

- Make a conscious effort to slow down and enjoy the moment.
- Use breathing techniques to slow down and find balance in your life.
- Use meditation or yoga to help you "slow down" and put your mind at ease.
- Control the Internet; don't let it control you.
- Escape from electronics at least 30 minutes every 3 to 4 hours.
- Listen to music, learn to paint or sew, try something new.
- Go for a walk— you can burn calories and reduce your stress at the same time.

Cited References

1. Zee, P. C., Attarian, H., & Videnovic, A. (2013). Circadian rhythm abnormalities. Continuum: Lifelong Learning in Neurology, 19(1 Sleep Disorders), 132–147.

2. Jabr, F. (2013, October 15). Why your brain needs more downtime. Scientific American. Retrieved from http://www.scientificamerican.com/article/mental-downtime/

3. Craig, R., Yaxley, V., Bridges, S., & Hawkins, V. (2014). Health Survey for England, NatCen. Retrieved from http://healthsurvey.hscic.gov.uk/support-guidance/public-health/health-survey-for-england-2013.aspx

4. Caruso, C. C. (2014). Negative impacts of shiftwork and long work hours. Rehabilitation Nursing, 39, 16-25.

5. Griep, R., Bastos, L. S., Fonseca, M., Silva-Costa, A., Portela, L., Toivanen, S. & Rotenberg, L. (2014). Years worked at night and body mass index among registered nurses from eighteen public hospitals in Rio de Janeiro, Brazil. BMC Health Services Research, 14, 603.

6. Jang, T., Kim, H. R., Lee, H. M., & Koo, J. W. (2013). Long work hours and obesity in korean adult workers. Journal of Occupational Health, 55, 359-366.

7. Au, N., Hauck, K. & Hollingsworth, B. (2013). Employment, work hours and weight gain among middle-aged women. International Journal of Obesity, 37, 718-724.

8. Corsica, J., Hood, M. M., Katterman, S., Kleinman, B. & Ivan, I. (2014). Development of a novel mindfulness and cognitive behavioral intervention for stress-eating: a comparative pilot study. Eating Behaviors, 15, 694-699.

9. Dalen, J., Smith, B. W., Shelley, B. M., Sloan, A. L., Leahigh, L. & Begay, D. (2010). Pilot study: mindful eating and living (MEAL): weight, eating behavior, and psychological outcomes associated with a mindfulness-based intervention for people with obesity. Complimentary Therapies in Medicine, 18, 260-264.

10. Johnson, D. C., Thom, N. J., Stanley, E. A., Haase, L., Simmons, A. N., Shih, P. A., Thompson, W. K., Potterat, E. G., Minor, T. R., & Paulus, M. P. (2014). Modifying resilience mechanisms in at-risk individuals: a

controlled study of mindfulness training in Marines preparing for deployment. American Journal of Psychiatry, 171(8), 844-853.

11. Peale, N. V. (1952). The power of positive thinking. NJ: Prentice-Hall.

12. Luders, E., Cherbuin, N., & Kurth F. (2015). Forever young(er): potential age-defying effects of long-term meditation on gray matter atrophy. Frontiers in Psychology. doi: 0.3389/fpsyg.2014.01551

13. Peters, R. (2006). Ageing and the brain. Postgraduate Medical Journal, 82(964), 84–88. doi:10.1136/pgmj.2005.036665

14. Fjell, A. M., Walhovd, K. B., Fennema-Notestine, C., McEvoy, L. K., Hagler, D. J., Holland, D., Brewer, J. B., & Dale, A. M. (2009). One-year brain atrophy evident in health aging. Journal of Neuroscience, 29(48), 15223-15231. doi: 10.1523/JNEUROSCI.3252-09.2009

15. Nyberg, L, Lo¨vde´n, M., Riklund, K., Lindenberger, U., & Ba¨ckman, L. (2012) Memory aging and brain maintenance. Trends in Cognitive Science, 16, 292–305.

16. Carlson, B. W., & Palmer, M. H. (2014). Nocturia in older adults: implications for nursing practice and aging in place. Nursing Clinics of North America, 49(2), 233-50. doi: 10.1016/j.cnur.2014.02.009

17. Black, D. S., O'Reilly, G. A., Olmstead, R., Breen, E. C., & Irwin, M. R. (2015). Mindfulness meditation and improvement in sleep quality and daytime impairment among older adults with sleep disturbances: a randomized clinical trial. JAMA Intern Medicine, 175(4), 494-501. doi: 10.1001/jamainternmed.2014.8081

18. Brendel, D. (2015, February). There are risks to mindfulness at work. Harvard Business Review. Retrieved from https://hbr.org/2015/02/there-are-risks-to-mindfulness-at-work

19. Yadav, R. K., Magan, D., Mehta, N., Sharma, R. & Mahapatra, S. C. (2012). Efficacy of a short-term yoga-based lifestyle intervention in reducing stress and inflammation: preliminary results. Journal of Alternative and Complementary Medicine, 18(7), 662-667. doi: 10.1089/acm.2011.0265

20. Rioux, J. G. & Ritenbaugh, C. (2013). Narrative review of yoga intervention clinical trials including weight-related outcomes. Alternative Therapies in Health and Medicine, 19, 32-46.

21. Manchanda, S. C. & Madan, K. (2014). Yoga and meditation in cardio-vascular disease. Clinical Research in Cardiology, 103, 675-680.

22. McCann, U. D., Penetar, D. M., Shaham, Y., Thorne, D. R., Gillin, J. C., Sing, H. C., Thomas, M. A., & Belenky, G. (1992). Sleep deprivation and impaired cognition: possible role of brain catecholamines. Biological Psychiatry, 31(11), 1082-1097.

23. Balkin, T. J., Kamimori, G. H., Redmond, D. P., Vigneulle, R. M., Thorne, D. R., Belenky, G, & Wesensten, N. J. (2004). On the importance of countermeasures in sleep and performance models. Aviation Space & Environmental Medicine, 75(S3), A155-157.

24. Sallinen, M., Härmä, M., Akerstedt, T., Rosa, R. & Lillqvist, O. (1998). Promoting alertness with a short nap during a night shift. Journal of Sleep Research, 7, 240-247.

25. Smith-Coggins, R., Howard, S. K., Mac, D. T., Wang, C., Kwan, S., Rosekind, M. R…Gaba, D. M. (2006). Improving alertness and performance in emergency department physicians and nurses: the use of planned naps. Annals of Emergency Medicine, 48, 596-604.

26. Schweitzer, P. K., Randazzo, A. C., Stone, K., Erman, M. & Walsh, J. K. (2006). Laboratory and field studies of naps and caffeine as practical countermeasures for sleep-wake problems associated with night work. Sleep, 29, 39-50.

27. Army Medicine. (2014). Performance triad: activity, nutrition and sleep. Retrieved from http://armymedicine.mil/Pages/performance-triad.aspx

28. Hancock, P., Szalma, J. L. (Eds.) (2008). Performance under stress. UK: Ashgate Publishing Limited.

29. Mednick, S. C. (2008). Take a nap! Change your life. New York, NY: Workman Publishing Company, Inc.

Additional Resources

Chu, P., Gotink, R. A., Yeh, G. Y., Goldie, S. J. & Hunink, M. M. (2014). The effectiveness of yoga in modifying risk factors of cardiovascular disease and metabolic syndrome: a systematic review and meta-analysis of randomized controlled trials. *European Journal of Preventive Cardiology. Dec. 15. pii: 2047487314562741*

Gindrat, A., Chytiris, M., Balerna, M., Rouiller, E. M. & Ghosh, A. (2015). Use-dependent cortical processing from fingertips in touchscreen phone users. *Cell, 25*, 109–115.

Han, K., Trinkoff, A. M., Storr, C. L. & Geiger-Brown, J. (2011). Job stress and work schedules in relation to nurse obesity. *Journal of Nursing Administration, 41*, 488-495.

Hemmingsson, E. (2014). A new model of the role of psychological and emotional distress in promoting obesity: conceptual review with implications for treatment and prevention. *Obesity Reviews, 15*, 769-779.

Kawada, Tomoyuki. (2014). Long working hours and obesity with special reference to sleep duration. *Journal of Occupation Health, 56*, 399-400.

Kivimäki, M., Virtanen, M., Kawachi, I., Nyberg, S. T., Alfredsson, L., Batty, G. D. ... Jokela, M. (2014). Long working hours, socioeconomic status, and the risk of incident type 2 diabetes: a meta-analysis of published and unpublished data from 222,120 individuals. *The Lancet Diabetes and Endocrinology, 3*, 27–34.

Milia, L. D., Vandelanotte, C. & Duncan, M. J. (2013). The association between short sleep and obesity after controlling for demographic, lifestyle, work and health related factors. *Sleep Medicine, 14*, 319-323.

Ramin, C., Devore, E. E., Wang, W., Pierre-Paul, J., Wegrzyn, L. R. & Schernhammar, E. S. (2014). Night shift work at specific age ranges and chronic disease risk factors. *Occupational and Environmental Medicine.* doi:10.1136/oemed-2014-102292

Rogers, A. E. & Aldrich, M. S. (1993). The effect of regularly scheduled naps on sleep attacks and excessive daytime sleepiness associated with narcolepsy. *Nursing Research and Practice, 42*, 111-117.

Solovieva, S., Lallukka, T., Virtanen, M. & Viikari-Juntura, E. (2013). Psychosocial factors at work, long work hours, and obesity: a systematic review. *Scandinavian Journal of Work, Environment, & Health, 39,* 241-258.

Spiers, K. E., Liechty, J. M. & Wu, C. F. (2014). Sleep, but not other daily routines, mediates the association between maternal employment and BMI for preschool children. *Sleep Medicine, 15,* 1590-1593.

4

Bringing It All Together

I hope you have enjoyed this material and have taken the time to think about each of the three main themes—eating, sleeping, and slowing down. It is important, because if you can manage these themes on a daily basis, I believe you will be able to live a healthier and longer life.

Of course, these three simple behaviors are not the full determinants of your longevity, but they do have a major role in the quality of your life.

Accept that you need to make some changes in your life and get started today; don't put it off. More than likely you have a family member or friend who needs to do it too, so give them a call to get them engaged.

Before you go off to run that marathon, make sure you complete the five tasks outlined below:

#1 – Get a Medical Check-Up

First, when was the last time you had a medical check-up? If it was recently, then look at your results. How did your weight compare to normal? Was your cholesterol within range? Did you have any results out of the ordinary? What did your healthcare provider suggest that you do?

If you haven't had a check-up, then get online or on the phone, and make an appointment. It really is important that you get a full physical examination before you embark on a life changing path. Granted, there isn't anything I have mentioned that should harm you, but remember the section on genes. There just might be something that you don't know about, and now isn't the time to find out.

#2 – Know Your Body Weight and Body Mass Index

Second, how does your body weight measure against age-appropriate norms? While it would be awesome if your body weight was close to your weight in high school, the likelihood of that just isn't realistic. How do you measure up? Are you underweight, overweight, or just about right? By the way, did you know that being underweight can cause health problems?

Now that you have accepted the status of your body weight, look up your body mass index (BMI). Calculate it using the link from the CDC: http://www.cdc.gov/healthyweight/assessing/bmi/adult_bmi/english_bmi_calculator/bmi_calculator.html0

Getting Started, Write It Down

So far, you have determined your medical health, and hopefully, there are no major issues requiring further investigation. You know your body weight, and you are ready to begin.

Now, get a spiral notebook or binder and write down the date. You have just solidified your inner goal to change your life. Way to go!

Next, summarize your feelings about your current health. Make note of your body weight, your health condition, and your cholesterol profile from your health records. What are your goals over the next one, three and twelve months? Remember, make them realistic, something that challenges but doesn't frustrate.

One more thing, go to the mirror and take a picture, just for you. It is best if you are naked or in a swim suit but follow your comfort level. Use this picture to help you when times are tough and when the temptation to go back to your old habits are strong.

Now let's get to the final three tasks.

#3 – Track Your Dietary Pattern

The third component of your get-started program is to find out how well you eat by writing it down in your notebook. While you are at it, determine when and why you eat. This is important because behavior drives a lot of our eating patterns and health outcomes. Do you eat late in the morning or, perhaps, late at night, after work, after the gym, or after night school? Do you eat when you are depressed? Does your medication make you eat, or, perhaps, not eat? These are all important questions that you need to understand so that you can manage and make changes to your diet.

Okay, so you have done all that stuff listed above. Now what? Well, for starters what did you eat? Did you succumb and eat that chocolate donut at work, or you ate ice cream after having an argument with your spouse or partner? Maybe you went one step further and had two bowls of ice cream. For most of us, we all have a tendency to gravitate to carbohydrates, so be careful.

#4 – Track Your Sleep

The fourth component of the program is to track your sleep. I bet you never knew how important sleep was to your health. I have presented

71

fairly solid evidence regarding the importance of sleep on glucose, obesity, and diabetes. It really is important to fully understand your sleep habits.

Honestly, there aren't a lot of great sleep books or programs to help you, and I have yet to see a decent smart phone application in this regard. The quantified sleep devices such as FitBit®, Jawbone®, and others are a step in the right direction, but I don't think you need to spend the money to track your sleep for this purpose.

For sleep, you need to log when you went to bed, how long it took you to fall asleep, when you got up, how many times you got up to go to the bathroom, and how you felt when you woke up (e.g., sleepy, groggy, peppy, energized)?

Now, overlay this sleep log with your daily activity calendar. Do you notice any patterns? Did watching that late night talk show make you go to bed later, which meant you got fewer hours of good, restful sleep? Did you drink alcohol or take medications that made you get up and go to the bathroom every few hours? Do certain activities, certain people, or certain days tend to precede poor sleep? It is important to know these sleep inhibitors, so that you can manage them better.

#5 – Track Your Quiet Time

Okay, we are almost done with the get started check list. You probably know by now that the last and final component is slowing down. Does the mention of doing nothing make you feel guilty?

Did you try the breathing exercise outlined in Chapter 3? Were you able to calm your mind, without thinking about work, family, or other stuff? Did you put aside some time today just for you? Did you take a few moments to relax and stretch? Did you say a favorite prayer or chant? Did you think about a loved one or a deceased family member? Did you push life out of your mind today, so you could have just a moment or two of silence or personal reflection?

Go to your notebook and write down the answers to these questions. Journal entry is perhaps one of the best ways to track and understand your behavior. You might even find that the process of writing helps you to slow down. What a great way to just let your mind wander and your thoughts to flow. Give it a try. What do you have to lose?

It is important to take the time for yourself, and while you are at it, make sure that you allow your loved ones and those around you to share in that experience as well.

Now, the Real Challenge Begins

The hardest part of change is getting started. So, if you have completed the check list, you are ready to embark on a life changing path toward better health and longevity. The material discussed in this book should give you confidence that you control much of your success.

As I finish this chapter and go to press, there is an editorial in the *British Journal of Sports Medicine* (1) that has been quite controversial. The three authors are leading experts in the field of sports medicine, nutrition, and exercise science, so their comments must not be taken lightly. I believe their statement, "you cannot outrun a bad diet," sums up their opinions quite nicely. Much to my delight, they provide solid evidence that the preponderance of food and the marketing of unhealthy food are the main reasons for the global obesity epidemic. They caution that exercise alone cannot override excessive caloric intake, which speaks to my point in Chapter 1. You need a concerted reduction in daily caloric intake and increased daily physical activity to burn off the excess energy stored as fat.

I leave you with one final concept that we touched upon in Chapter 1, which is "energy in = energy out." Once you have achieved your ideal body weight, if you can keep that equation balanced, you should be able to maintain your body weight for life.

I wish you good fortune and success on your journey to better health and longevity. I hope that this information has been helpful and instructive for you. Also, don't forget to share this message with the world.

Cited References

1. Malhotra, A., Noakes, T., & Phinney, S. (2015) It is time to bust the myth of physical inactivity and obesity: you cannot outrun a bad diet. British Journal of Sports Medicine. Advance online publication. doi: 10.1136/bjsports-2015-094911

Thank you for reading my book.

I want to thank my family for their support and especially my wife, Kristee Emens-Hesslink, for editing, proofreading, and her ever thoughtful insights. In addition, I want to thank my friends and colleague, who helped guide me to the final manuscript.

If you enjoyed reading my book, please take the time to post a comment on my Facebook page: www.facebook.com/eatlessandsleepmore?ref=hl

And, don't forget to write a comment at your favorite retailer.

Sincerely,
Robert

About the Author

Robert has spent a lifetime trying to understand human metabolism and weight management. As a young boy, he struggled with his weight and the burden of being overweight. His interest in sports lead him to study exercise science and sports medicine, eventually, earning a Doctorate of Science from Sargent College of Health Sciences, Boston University, Massachusetts. Robert served as a Naval Officer in the United States Navy for six years. He conducted research on human performance in environmental extremes as a research physiologist in the Medical Services Corps. Upon leaving the United States Navy, Robert served in a variety of positions within the nutritional supplement and medical foods industry.

For the past two decades, Robert has incorporated his passion and knowledge about healthy living into his wealth management practice. Robert counsels individuals and business owners on how to best incorporate wellness and wealth into their lives.

www.centerpointeadvisers.com

Coming Soon

How to Manage Your Health for Better Wealth

by Robert L. Hesslink, Jr., Sc.D., Ch.F.C.

This new book is inspired by the many readers of *Eat Less, Sleep More, and Slow Down*, who wanted more help, more guidance, and a plan. *Eat Less, Sleep More, and Slow Down*, offered the story behind the biology and nutrition of better health, *How to Manage Your Health for Better Wealth* will help the reader understand the 'why' in "Why should I change my behavior?"

The book reviews the main topics presented in Dr. Hesslink's first book and elaborates on additional material that plays a role in wellness and wealth. Each chapter reviews new science and outlines the financial cost of waiting to change. In addition, the book includes a plan to help the reader track, monitor, and analyze how achieving better health, leads to better wealth.

CPSIA information can be obtained
at www.ICGtesting.com
Printed in the USA
FSOW03n0541190217
30842FS